Sacrificial Lambs

Sacrificial
Lambs

A Liberal Reporter Exposes How the Progressive Left
Harms Children in the Name of Gender Ideology

Anita Bartholomew

PITCHSTONE PUBLISHING
DURHAM, NORTH CAROLINA

Pitchstone Publishing
Durham, North Carolina
www.pitchstonebooks.com

Library of Congress Cataloging-in-Publication Data

Names: Bartholomew, Anita author
Title: Sacrificial lambs : a liberal reporter exposes how the progressive
    left harms children in the name of gender ideology / Anita Bartholomew.
Description: Durham, North Carolina : Pitchstone Publishing, [2025] |
    Includes bibliographical references. | Summary: "Today, more than 1 in
    20 teens say they are transgender or gender questioning-an order of
    magnitude higher than just a decade ago. How is it possible that so many
    youngsters-within just a matter of years-became persuaded that they'd
    been born in the wrong bodies? As Anita Bartholomew reveals in
    Sacrificial Lambs, following her multiyear investigation into the
    phenomenon, the answer lies not with gender-confused children but rather
    with our most trusted institutions and the adults who run them: the
    medical professionals who "transition" children to facsimiles of the
    opposite sex before they are old enough to know what sex is; the
    teachers who tell kindergarteners that doctors only "guessed" their sex
    at birth; and the mainstream media outlets that label chemical and
    surgical experiments on children as "life-saving" care. Exposing the
    ideology's roots, trunk, branches, and means of pollination, she
    uncovers a committed, well-funded, multi-faction gender coalition that
    victimizes vulnerable children, teens, and young adults. She also
    explains why so many mental health professionals, educators, and
    government officials themselves became deeply invested in promoting and
    perpetuating gender ideology. Backed up by an array of peer-reviewed
    studies, statistics, court documents, and first-hand accounts from
    experts and those directly affected, Sacrificial Lambs shows that every
    argument you've heard in favor of gender ideology is wrong"— Provided
    by publisher.
Identifiers: LCCN 2025020714 (print) | LCCN 2025020715 (ebook) | ISBN
    9781634312745 paperback | ISBN 9781634312752 ebook
Subjects: LCSH: Gender identity in children—United States | Gender
    transition—Moral and ethical aspects—United States | Children—United
    States—Social conditions
Classification: LCC HQ18.55 .B37 2025 (print) | LCC HQ18.55 (ebook)
LC record available at https://lccn.loc.gov/2025020714
LC ebook record available at https://lccn.loc.gov/2025020715

Contents

Introduction   7

1. The Myth of the Magical Child   21
2. Consent to This "Care" . . . or Else   44
3. The Media and the Message   60
4. Today's Lesson: Reject Your Sex   76
5. Watch Out Kids, Your Parents Aren't "Safe"   96
6. Watch Out Parents: No One,
      Nowhere, and Nothing Is Safe   117
7. Is Transgender Actually a Thing
      (and Is It Just One Thing)?   137
8. Males in Girls' Sports—How Is This Fair?   157
9. Why Are We Letting Males Invade
      Female-Only Spaces?   176
10. Why Have We All Gone Mad?   195
11. It's Time to Reclaim Reality and Sanity   216

Acknowledgments   230
Appendix I: The Effects and Limits
      of Trump's Executive Orders   232
Appendix II: Advice to Parents   237
Resources   244
Notes   246
About the Author

Introduction

"A man who lies to himself, and believes his own lies, becomes unable to recognize truth, either in himself or in anyone else."

—Fyodor Dostoyevsky, *The Brothers Karamazov*

Until recent years, I had mostly used gender-confused people's "preferred pronouns." It seemed rude not to. Living in the uber-progressive Pacific Northwest, I'd met a number of people who considered themselves trans. They didn't seem to be bothering anyone else.

So, if I referred to a man who identified as a woman as "she," it seemed no worse than what I'd do if a child invited me to a tea party with imaginary tea. I'd pretend-drink the pretend-tea.

I thought: Where's the harm?

Like many other people, I assumed trans was the new gay. I bought into the oft-repeated claim that "transwomen" were the "most vulnerable members of our society." Taking that as gospel, I was careful about what I said and what I did around people who identified as trans.

I thought I was being kind.

I can pinpoint the moment when I first recognized there was something not quite right about all this.

I was at a holiday party, standing in my friends' dining room, sipping a glass of red wine, next to a guy wearing black pumps and a black and pink flowered dress who I'd met on a number of similar occasions. I found myself effusively complimenting him on his new hair color. As I did, I became conscious, almost as if I were a third party standing apart and watching this interaction, that I was play-acting. I didn't find him or his hair all that interesting. I wouldn't have said much more than hello if he were dressed in men's clothing. I was giving him the kind of exaggerated attention I'd give a little girl who'd wandered into a roomful of adults to show off her doll, stopping whatever I was doing to ask the doll's name. I was treating this guy who was half a foot taller than I and probably had fifty pounds on me like a fragile child.

This was a grown man. He knew he was a man. I knew he was a man. And he was wearing the most elaborately feminine outfit of any guest in the room.

Though I realized I'd behaved in an odd, preprogrammed way, my negative feelings had to do with my own play-acting, not with his.

It didn't dawn on me until much later that my behavior was much like that of all the other liberals I knew, and reflected the messages society was getting from virtually all our major institutions.

At the time, I'd had no intention of writing about the trans phenomenon, and when I began to, a few years later, it was almost by accident. I'd been researching the woke racial movement. It seemed both troubling and comical that so many of my friends and colleagues were trying to outdo each other in self-castigation for having committed the sin of being born white. I looked into where all this was coming from and found it in best-selling books my friends and colleagues were reading. I also found it in what children were being taught in school: if they were born white, they were oppressors, essentially beyond redemption. And if they were born black, they were doomed to be oppressed forever, with no hope of escape. Talk about a noxious message!

As I investigated further, gender ideology and the broader umbrella it falls under, queer theory, kept popping up, uninvited. Racial and gender identity were being treated as intertwined social justice issues. This wasn't the social justice movement of my youth, of crusading for peace and for the rights of the downtrodden. The current-day concept of social justice required that people be treated *un*justly if they happened to be the wrong "identity," downtrodden or not.

The wrong identities included members of the "cis-heteropatriarchy" (heterosexual, and *not* gender-confused—with points deducted for being male). I soon discovered that queer theory counts all "sexual minorities" as marginalized victims. Though that includes anyone who identifies as transgender or gay, it doesn't stop there. Anyone whose sexual proclivities tended toward the deviant were *also* considered marginalized and in need of support from social justice warriors. Yes, even those whose sexual tastes run to the illegal.

While looking into the racially charged lessons taught in left-leaning school districts, I discovered that teachers, prompted by materials from queer theory–inspired sexuality education organizations such as SIECUS, Advocates for Youth, Planned Parenthood, and others, were telling kids that doctors had only guessed what sex the kids were at birth. Their body parts didn't actually determine whether they were boys or girls, though. They might be either. Or both. Or neither. From the time children in the most progressive school districts walked through the front door, they were bombarded with messages saying that they could ditch their sex and choose another.

This was next-level nuts indoctrination. And it got worse as they got older. By fourth or fifth grade, sexuality educators would be teaching them that they could avoid going through the "wrong puberty" by taking powerful drugs that block puberty's onset—and also block the skeletal and brain development that occurs during puberty, potentially permanently.

Nonprofit social justice organizations also distributed materials for schools to use in instruction. The "Black Lives Matter 13 Principles for Schools," for example, included an affirmation about "freeing ourselves from the tight grip of cis-heteropatriarchal assumptions" and told kids to "do the work required to dismantle cisgender privilege."

Almost all schools in districts that leaned even slightly left celebrated Pride month. In the most progressive, Pride flags and other transgender swag adorned the bulletin boards, walls, and windows year-round.

How was all this affecting children?

I realized that I already had the beginnings of an answer when I thought of all my friends and colleagues whose kids had announced, without prior warning, that they were no longer their actual sex: the gay son of my close friends in Portland . . . the granddaughter of a man in my Oregon City philosophy discussion group . . . the niece of a colleague in Orlando . . . a teen member of my extended family in Hoboken . . . both the son and daughter of a friend in San Jose . . . and, in my Austin friend's family, three out of four grandchildren.

Just in my small social circle, I could see a burgeoning epidemic. But, of course, it wasn't just my social circle. It was all over the country.

Scratch that. It was all over what's loosely labeled the "free world." Canada. Mexico. The United Kingdom. Finland. France. Italy. Australia. New Zealand. Germany. Belgium. Spain. The Netherlands. And beyond.

It might be quicker to list the places that haven't been affected.

This was a much more compelling issue than the woke racial movement.

It also dramatically answered what I'd assumed was a rhetorical question:

Where's the harm?

If I was willing to call a man "she," I would have little credibility when I protested a fourteen-year-old girl getting her breasts cut off . . . or a seventeen-year-old boy having his penis sliced open, hollowed out, and inverted.

But this never happens, right? So, no one needs to be concerned. If there were any doubt, the country's most prominent gender surgeon, Dr. Marci Bowers, a man who identifies as a woman, assured viewers in 2023 on *Face the Nation* that reports of youngsters undergoing gender surgeries are unfounded:

> *Surgery really is not done under the age of eighteen, except in severe cases, usually top surgery for trans masculine persons. And even that is rare, I think the estimates are something like fifty-seven surgeries under the age of eighteen were done for trans individuals.*

Without a national registry of medical procedures, it's impossible to document how many such surgeries have been done in the United States. But researchers, relying on gender identity disorder–related and sex reassignment codes in two hospital databases, published estimates of gender surgeries performed over just four years, from 2016 to 2020. While their estimates are necessarily an undercount, they found that among those twelve to eighteen years old, 405 had undergone genital surgery and 3,215 had had breast surgery.

Among those 405 genital surgeries that, according to Bowers, simply are not done, was one televised on the reality TV series *I Am Jazz*. In that show, a seventeen-year-old boy had his penis sliced open, hollowed out, and inverted.

That surgery was performed by Dr. Marci Bowers.

No one has ever been able to accurately predict which children with the formerly rare gender identity disorder that begins in very early childhood will persist in their desire to be the opposite sex. Depending on the study, it might be anywhere from 10 to about 20 percent, but a recent analysis suggests it's likely much closer to the lower end of the spectrum. That means that, from the outset, medically transitioning children was always fated to do great harm. It was always fated to mutilate the healthy bodies of children who would have otherwise grown up to accept their bodies, typically as gay and bisexual adults.

It was impossible for it to be otherwise.

So why would anyone do it?

One of the first things you'll learn as you read *Sacrificial Lambs* is that the research touted to support pharmaceutical and surgical interventions to allow kids to mimic the opposite sex was fatally flawed. Researchers made a series of honest mistakes. But they also made reckless assumptions. And they ignored earlier research that contradicted what they wanted to believe was true. After the worst of the research errors were discovered, the headlines should have screamed "Stop everything!" And everything should have stopped.

We're talking about children, after all. No one would charge full steam ahead on damaging the healthy bodies of children on the basis of faulty research. Right?

Wrong.

Here in the United States and in Europe, those error-laden studies continued to be lauded in both scientific circles and the popular press. The corrections, meanwhile, were buried. Gender researchers continued to search for good evidence that puberty blockers, cross-sex hormones, and mutilating surgeries were helping gender-confused kids. They never found it. Whether due to wishful thinking or deception or both, they kept claiming they had.

But at first, few children were affected. Trans was not yet a craze. It *was* a fascination, though—something so utterly bizarre that people could only gawk and nod along as activists and gender physicians (who were, too often, one and the same) explained what they thought they knew. When the 2013 *Diagnostic and Statistical Manual of Mental Disorders, Fifth Edition* (DSM-5), was published, those who identified as trans were still rare. Adolescent-onset was virtually unheard of. The DSM-5 authors estimated that between 0.005% to 0.014% (five to fourteen in 100,000) of adult males with onset at any age, and between 0.002% to 0.003% (two to three in 100,000) of females suffered from "gender dysphoria" (originally and more accurately called "gender identity disorder," but renamed for the sole purpose of reducing stigma).

What those involved in facilitating social, medical, and surgical transition thought they knew was that gender-confused people committed suicide at alarming rates. But this, too, was based on flawed data, as you'll read in chapter 2. You couldn't even call it data. Two anonymous internet surveys, promoted by trans activists online, asked respondents, among other questions, whether they'd considered suicide. A large percentage said they had. Gender specialists used these responses to persuade parents to consent to extreme and irreversible medical and surgical procedures on their children with the question: "Would you rather have a live son or a dead daughter?" When faced with such a choice, parents often gave in—to devastating effect.

But even the unreliable survey responses didn't support the claim that "transitioning" prevented self-harm. If anything, as you'll see in later chapters, kids set on the trans path grew increasingly unstable.

As pediatric gender clinics sprang up around the country, that extortionist question was asked tens of thousands of times. All the major medical associations got on board the trans train, each apparently assuming that there was good evidence for treating children with chemicals that did monstrous things to their bodies. They believed that the treatments were "life-saving." There was no good evidence. None. Nothing.

After a huge scandal in the United Kingdom that showed that children were being rushed into treatment, the country's National Health Service (NHS) commissioned a review of all the evidence gender specialists were relying on to decide to "transition" children and found it was more likely hurting than helping. Reviews by Finland and Sweden found much the same.

The American public was mostly in the dark about all this. You might assume that this would be an enormous scandal. And it would have been, if our mainstream media reported accurately about any of it. As you'll see in chapter 3, however, media kept touting the non-existent benefits of "gender-affirming care" for teens, and ran story after story about how state governments that restricted these procedures were putting children's health and even their very lives at risk. With rare exceptions, whenever CNN, NPR, the *New York Times*, the *Washington Post*, or any local mainstream media outlets mention opposition to transgender ideology, it's either openly stated or indirectly implied that such opposition comes exclusively from radical bigots. Transphobes. Knuckle-dragging Neanderthals.

By 2017, the Williams Institute of UCLA estimated that 0.7 percent (700 of 100,000) of kids thirteen to seventeen openly identified as the wrong sex—an exponential increase over just four years. By 2022, the Williams Institute had to revise its estimates upward to twice that: 1.4 percent of thirteen- to seventeen-year-olds.

One year later, in 2023, a survey by the Centers for Disease Control found that 5.5 percent of high school students either said they were trans or thought they might be.

Look at how those numbers grew over a relatively short period. From a maximum of 14 in 100,000 in the total population back in 2013 to almost 6 in 100 kids in just ten years. As more school systems adopt queer theory–focused sexuality education programs each year, expect those numbers to continue to rise.

If this craze hasn't yet affected your family, odds are that it will. It might be your child, your niece, your nephew, your grandchild, or the kid down the street who babysat for your little ones over the summer.

As you'll see in chapter 4, the above figures don't even account for all those under the age of thirteen who might not yet spend much time on the internet but are being indoctrinated right now, in their schools, by the very people parents should be able to trust the most.

You'll meet children in these pages who at ten, eleven, or twelve years old were being told by their teachers, and by contractors hired by school systems to teach sex ed, that they might be trapped in the wrong bodies.

Youngsters who are lonely, who don't fit in, who are awkward, who have mental health problems, who've suffered trauma, begin to imagine that it's because they really *are* the wrong sex. They might have felt like misfits before, but they're love-bombed when they come out. "Trans" kids are cool kids.

With broad societal acceptance of trans ideology, leading to queer theory–tinged lessons becoming the norm in the classrooms of liberal democracies, other countries also have been seeing rapidly increasing numbers of the gender-confused. Referrals to the United Kingdom's single pediatric gender clinic increased by 4,400 percent in girls over eight years; boys asking for gender treatment increased by 1,646 percent. Sweden, Spain, the Netherlands, Finland, and others have similar numbers to report.

Queer theory got into K–12 schools the same way it got into so many other institutions: via those who were steeped in it at their colleges and universities. Upon getting their degrees, these indoctrinated grads fanned out into their chosen professions and brought the ideology with them.

Queer theory's outrageous concepts, which we'll explore in-depth shortly, filtered down to the rest of us as received wisdom. Doctors, therapists, teachers, journalists, politicians, publishers, entertainers, and the majority of our most distinguished institutions and nonprofits began treating baseless trans advocacy as unassailable Truth. Reality TV and other entertainment promoted it. Wherever you looked, trans was in.

If we'd thought about what these presumed experts were telling us, we'd have realized that none of it made sense. How could a large share of the kids in a middle school classroom today imagine they were the wrong sex, when fifteen, twenty or more years ago, it was unlikely you'd have come across even student confused about his or her sex? Other than in cases of paraphilias that involve cross-dressing and might begin early, never before was there such a thing as an adolescent-onset gender identity disorder. It simply didn't occur. Prior to the current mass psychogenic event (the technical term for an imagined condition that spreads from person to person), the rare cases of gender confusion that occurred in girls almost always began in early childhood. Think toddler age. And childhood-onset gender identity disorder almost always *resolved* in adolescence—it didn't suddenly appear then.

If any other affliction had suddenly struck a population of youngsters who had never before been susceptible to it, there would be a massive attempt to find the reasons and reverse it. Instead, there's been a massive attempt by those who socially or monetarily gain from transitioning children to promote and celebrate it—and to punish anyone who tries to stand in the way.

As you'll see in succeeding chapters, the rainbows-and-unicorns version of queer theory taught in left-leaning school districts across the country gets more graphic and more highly sexualized as kids get older. They're told that in addition to identifying out of their sex, they might be pansexual or polyamorous. While the slides and other curricular materials I've reviewed often just have bullet points that don't tell the whole story of what's discussed in such classes, when girls get the idea they can identify as gay boys, and boys imagine they can be lesbians, it's apparent that some kids are being taught that sexually, anything goes. This kind of instruction happens before children are developmentally mature enough to grasp what sexuality even is.

Depending on the school system, the extreme focus on sex can begin as early as kindergarten. In some of the most progressive schools, children are taught to memorize vocabulary words like "vulva," "scrotum," and "clitoris" about the same time they're learning more typical vocabulary words like "school," "cat," and "dog." The words they're taught not to use? Boy and girl. Gendered language is considered disrespectful to those who are gender-confused.

By fourth grade sex ed class, under the guise of a puberty lesson, some children are being shown extremely graphic depictions of genitalia. School libraries promote books that qualify as porn, with images depicting people having gay and straight sex. Some schools even secretly provide breast binders and packers (to give the appearance of a cross-sex genital bulge) to girls. Boys can get tuckers (to minimize male genitalia).

When parents discover what's going on and try to protect their children, they're shunned, called transphobes, radical rightwingers—even though most are liberals and moderates. But it's an effective tactic to ensure that no other liberals or moderates will listen to them.

And then, of course, if the parents won't comply with the school's gender agenda, sometimes, the school calls Child Protective Services.

If you're an old-school liberal like me, you probably realize by now that none of what I've described above is liberal. Sexualizing children . . . refusing to let parents know that their children have been "transitioned" at school . . . turning children against their "unsafe" parents . . . threatening parents with the loss of their parental rights if they don't go along? This is authoritarian. It's tyrannical. It's cult-like.

The problem is that, if you consider yourself liberal or moderate, you probably have no idea that any of this is going on. The people who have been reporting on the excesses of gender ideology are mostly politically far to the right. In our polarized society, we refuse to listen to the people who our political tribe considers dead wrong on virtually everything. So, even when those wrong, wrong, wrong rightwingers absolutely nail the issue, we liberals have no clue. We can't hear them. And if their message somehow gets through, we won't believe them. It doesn't help that some who have written about the threat of gender ideology to children have equated queer theory with Marxism. That makes it easier for liberals and moderates to dismiss whatever they have to say. And that sets up those who are left of center to be blindsided when their kids are the targets.

This is the reason why I felt so passionately that this book's cover should identify me as a liberal. Most liberals will ignore anything from the rightwing. But no one can credibly call me rightwing. On most issues, I'm politically somewhat to the left of Vermont Senator Bernie Sanders.

Gender ideology shouldn't be a left or right issue. But since the progressive left has championed it, a dissenting voice sounding the alarm from the left might be the only one most liberals can hear.

There are those who brush off the threat of gender ideology, insisting it affects only a small portion of the population. But it affects all of us, even those who don't notice. It's altering society in obvious and more subtle ways. According to a 2023 poll, between 33 and 44 percent of

Americans, depending on age group, believe that "misgendering" someone (correctly identifying the person's sex) should be a criminal offense. We have a First Amendment that should protect us from such impulses but in some locales, including New York City, they're writing laws to punish people who correctly name a person's sex, anyway.

In other countries—Iceland, the United Kingdom, Spain, Mexico, Canada, Germany, and elsewhere—where there is no First Amendment protection, people actually *are* being imprisoned, or threatened with prison, for failing to comply with gender ideologues language demands.

When an entire culture agrees to deny biology and depart from reality, it becomes impossible to predict or control the consequences.

Make-believe is starting to make the rules. It's making rules for you, right now, whether you're aware of it or not. Government officials have been taking our willingness to pretend along as a sign that they should cement unreality into regulations and laws that we will now be forced to live by that penalize us for noticing what sex a person is. What happens next, if we continue to go along without complaint, is anyone's guess.

When I began my investigation, I was most concerned about the countless children being induced to imagine they might be trapped in the wrong bodies. I believed at first that adults were in a different category. To get shocked out of my assumptions required connecting with a great many young adults who had fallen for the false claim that they could change sex, some who have since detransitioned and some who still call themselves trans. Several detransitioners were gung ho on living the transgender life, right up to the epiphanic moment that they recognized it had all been a lie. It often emotionally devastated them—a devastation almost as profound as what they'd agreed to have done to their bodies.

These are the true "most vulnerable members of our society," the children and young adults who believed the lies. They are the sacrificial lambs on the altar of a movement that has no basis in fact or common sense. You'll meet some of them shortly.

Most people are also unaware that the gender make-believe sold to young people is driven, in large part, by adult sexual fantasies and fetishes.

No one promoting the ideology mentions the fetishists. Most activists refuse to admit they exist. But the majority of men now identifying as the opposite sex aren't what the average person imagines them to be. Mental health experts who study the phenomenon estimate that about three-quarters of the men claiming to identify as women are acting out the extreme sexual deviance of a paraphilia or fetish. Though transgenderism has been sold to the public as the new gay, most of these men, especially the ones who adopt their new identities in middle age or older, are heterosexual, not gay. They are straight men who are both attracted to women *and* get off sexually by imagining themselves to be women.

The average "transwoman," then, is a transvestic fetishist or autogynephile, often shortened to AGP (experts are divided on which men fall into each of these two deviant sexual categories, so you'll often see the terms transvestic fetishist and AGP used together, throughout). They dress in women's wear, become sexually aroused as they watch themselves in the mirror, and masturbate to that fantasy. Although cross-dressers like this have always been with us, they've almost always been closeted.

Today, this fetishism has been invited out of the dark corners. It's more than just normalized. It's catered to, treated with utmost deference. Celebrated. This is where we are now.

Public fetishism, under a pastel rainbow banner, is remaking our society.

When these fetishists come out of the closet, they usually claim to have been "born this way." They deny that their fetishes are fetishes, instead claiming a lifelong hidden female identity. That only makes sense if there are children who identify as the opposite sex—proof that people can be "born this way." If a child can be born in the wrong body, a grown man can claim he was once just such a child. And when he "comes out" as a woman, and society accepts him on his say-so, what happens next?

He's a woman. He gets access to all that is reserved for women and girls. He's in the shower stall next to your teenage daughter at the gym. He's the "sales lady" in the department store fitting room, helping women find a comfortable bra.

He's living his fetish, loud and proud, and no one dares to say he can't, unless they want to risk being ostracized, sued, or worse.

With his larger, stronger body, he's also winning medals in girls' and women's sports.

Males have taken over female sports at every level, from the playground to the Olympic arena. In K–12 sports, stronger, faster boys are taking girls' spots on teams. That means some girls will never get to play. When they do, they're often forced to undress in front of boys who claim female gender identities. The girls won't get the sports scholarships they worked so hard to qualify for throughout their school years if a male shows up in their sport. He might not have been fast enough or skilled enough to qualify for the boys' team but he can run circles around anyone on the girls'.

At the elite end of the spectrum, the United Nations Special Rapporteur on Violence Against Women and Girls reported that in more than 400 competitions in twenty-nine different sports, more than 600 female athletes lost 890 medals to males competing in female categories.

Statistics tell us that almost half of the male prisoners in federal penitentiaries claiming trans identities and demanding to the placed in women's prisons are sex offenders. This isn't an anomaly. Canada found much the same. So have other countries.

Male sex offenders have also claimed to be trans on numerous occasions to get lighter sentences. You'll learn just how well that worked out for them—and how badly it worked out for the women they're incarcerated with.

Women prisoners are being harassed, beaten, and raped by men who, by simply claiming to identify as female, are being locked into cells with them. You're about to learn more than anyone should ever have to know about this travesty.

Sacrificial Lambs is based on rock-solid evidence, thoroughly documented, showing that every argument you might have heard in favor of embracing gender ideology is false. Even if you're still a believer now, by the last page, after you've seen the breadth and depth of how gender ideology harms, not just our young, but all of society—you included—you should be ready to detox. This book is meant to help you do that.

We can't protect kids until we adults cure ourselves of any illusions that this is just another passing fad, a fringe movement that affects very few and will dissipate on its own. Gender ideology has a committed, well-funded, multi-faction army promoting and defending it. It's going to take the equivalent on the other side to stand up against it.

It seeped into our society because we didn't take its threat seriously. It seemed to require only this from us: that we be kind.

We couldn't have imagined that doctors would eagerly prescribe experimental drugs to mentally ill kids who fell for the make-believe, calling those chemicals "medically necessary" and "life-saving." We never expected our most trusted news sources to lie to us about what was happening. We couldn't guess that so many youngsters who "transitioned" would later look at their broken bodies and mourn.

We couldn't have predicted any of this. We didn't know.

But now, we do. At least, some of us do.

So, now it's time to be part of the solution—and reverse course.

Chapter 1

The Myth of the Magical Child

"I knew who I was this morning,
but I've changed a few times since then."

—Alice, in *Alice's Adventures in Wonderland*

I was probably ten or eleven years old when I learned in catechism class about the various stages that Catholic nuns went through on their way to becoming full-fledged members of the convent. The sister teaching the class told us that God calls the ones he wants. This wasn't something you just decided to do on your own. There were lots of steps and tests to ensure that your calling was real. The newbie nuns were postulates. Get past that stage and you progress to novice and finally, after some hazily described but important steps, you'd become a bride of Christ.

Like a lot of little Catholic girls, I was fascinated by all this. For a while, it seemed romantic, in its way. And there was that challenge: you've got to prove that God called you.

Well, I've always loved a challenge. My scheming little self was pretty sure I could either prove I'd been called or else fake it.

So, at ten or eleven, I toyed with the idea that this could be my future. If, at the time, you'd tried to warn me off by telling me I'd be giving up precious pieces of the life of a modern women—I'd never become a mother; I'd never even have sex; and my career would be chosen for me by the clergy—those wouldn't have been deterrents. To the adult me, sure, these would be dealbreakers. But I had no reference points for any of this back then. I was a child. None of those issues was on my radar.

I did wonder whether nuns still got their periods. I knew by then that the uterus shed its lining each month if it wasn't employed in cradling an implanted fetus. Maybe, I thought, God stopped nuns from menstruating, once they were "married" to him. They weren't ever going to have babies, so why would they need any of that?

I wasn't bold enough to ask about this potential fringe benefit, but I did wonder.

The lessons about nuns being married to God were given by a very appealing young woman who'd made the grade and who looked almost exotic in her crisp black and white habit. Was a marriage to a real live man better than one to a magical being? I had no reason to think so. Nunhood, if that's even a word, seemed faintly glamorous and certainly saintly.

It was around that same time that I met my new stepbrother, Davey. He was two years older than I was and seemed lightyears more knowledgeable and experienced. I'd never met anyone so smart before.

We'd stay up on the nights I slept over at my father's house, him in the top bed of the bunkbed and me on the one below, talking for hours when we were supposed to be going to sleep. He introduced me to philosophy, which didn't jibe with the Catholicism I'd learned in catechism classes. He challenged my religious schooling. If God could do anything, he asked, can he build a mountain so big that even he couldn't move it? A trick question, but an interesting one to preteen me. It proved that the nuns were wrong when they said the Almighty was, well, almighty. God actually did have limits, didn't he?

By thirteen or fourteen, thanks to those long-past-bedtime conversations with Davey, I'd started calling myself an atheist.

Even if my new stepbrother had never become part of my life, this was the trajectory my mind, as it developed, was destined to be on. Logic would eventually become more compelling than magic, despite the latter's charms. Had I succumbed to magic first, and taken those Catholic vows, it would have made life as a nun extremely inconvenient once I'd matured.

I was a precocious youngster. Adults always commented on my apparent maturity. They were wrong about that. I wasn't mature. Articulate, and probably quite poised for my age, I was no less a kid than any other kid (though my kid self would be offended by her adult self's assessment).

So why am I telling you all this? Because organized religions aren't the only ones that beguile children with promises of escape into an entirely different reality. I might have stayed fascinated long enough to enter the convent. But by the time I was mature enough to recognize my mistake, I wouldn't have damaged my body, mind, and perhaps even shortened my lifespan by taking powerful chemicals to cosmetically approximate something I wasn't. And I'd still have all the body parts I went in with.

Now it's your turn. Think back to when you were ten, or eleven, or twelve. Are you the same in every way as you were then? What's changed? If you could somehow tumble through time, back into the mind of that preteen you, and someone asked you the following questions, how would you answer?

What do you imagine your future will look like?

What scares you?

Whose opinion of you matters more than anyone else's?

What's your biggest secret?

What's your greatest shame?

After you've ruminated on these questions for a bit, consider yourself as you are today. And ask your adult self this:

How many of the decisions that will affect the rest of your life are you willing to delegate—right now—to that kid-version of you?

Pontificators about the goodness and necessity of so-called gender-affirming care for children seem never to consider that kids see life's possibilities differently. Their child-brains process information differently.

Children's brains aren't adult brains. Even after the rest of the body appears full-grown, the brain is still immature, still developing the complex connections in the prefrontal cortex that help adults plan, assess risks, and make decisions. That process isn't complete until sometime in our mid-twenties.

And that's the crux of the issue, isn't it? If you wouldn't let a kid make potentially devastating choices for *you*, based on a kid's limited understanding of how the world works, why would you cheer the idea of letting a kid make such irreversible decisions for him or herself?

An *Atlantic* article that ran in 2019 was headlined "Young Trans Children Know Who They Are." As the article reported, that was the conclusion of psychologist Kristina Olson, PhD, who'd studied children aged three to twelve who wanted to be the opposite sex—and whose parents went along with the children's desires. These families let their children use cross-sex pronouns, as well as dress as the opposite sex and sometimes take opposite-sex first names. With these changes, the children were said to have "socially transitioned."

The psychologist followed up after a number of years and found that almost all the children who had socially transitioned continued to identify out of their sex as they grew. Comparing them to children who merely showed non-stereotypical behavior for their sex, she found the latter group still content to be the girls and boys they were born to be.

Olson concluded that this meant there really was something different about the socially transitioned children. The kids "knew who they were" and who they were was not what their bodies said they were. They were actually a different gender. And most of them were going to "transition" completely as they grew. The article also pointed out that, per Olson's previous research, "children who are supported and affirmed in their transitions are just as mentally healthy as cisgender peers." Depression levels of the socially transitioned children were no different from that of children who weren't identifying out of their sex, and anxiety levels were only minimally elevated, according to her analysis. These findings were significant because earlier research consistently found such children suffered substantially higher rates of both anxiety and depression. The implication was that by "affirming," i.e., embracing their child's cross-sex identity, parents were acting in the best interests of the child's mental health.

Some of the children were already on puberty blockers to keep them from developing the typical traits of boys and girls as they matured into teens. Once on puberty blockers, almost all would eventually take cross-sex hormones and some would get genital surgeries and mastectomies to better mimic the opposite sex.

Olson's research results remarkably differed from those of earlier researchers who found that about 90 percent of gender-confused children naturally shed their gender distress around puberty (although an analysis of earlier research by MIT philosophy professor Alex Byrne shows that that's a conservative number; by adulthood, hardly any still suffered gender confusion). The author of the *Atlantic* article mentioned just one of these earlier studies, done in the Netherlands, which showed that almost all of the 127 children referred to a Dutch clinic for gender confusion eventually grew out of their gender confusion. Yet, that study's findings aligned with Olson's in one key respect: the few kids in the study who socially transitioned at a young age continued to claim a cross-sex identity as adolescents.

The implication of this finding should have been obvious: what set apart the children who stayed on the "trans" path was not the magical gender identity of the kids. It was the acquiescence of the grown-ups in their lives.

The grown-ups went along with the fantasy that these children were a different sex.

Children love to play make-believe. They might be a cowpoke one day, a surfer the next, an astronaut after that. Even when we adults play along with the game, eventually the game ends and the child is told to brush his teeth, get into his jammies, and go to bed.

But what happens when the game never ends? A little boy claims to be a girl. Everyone goes along with this, and he is never told to get out of costume. His parents don't just dress him as a girl. They call him by a girl's name. They introduce him as their daughter. They get him toys that girls typically play with but none of those that typically appeal to boys. Wouldn't that cement his "female" identity in his mind? Why wouldn't he continue to call himself a girl, when everything and everyone in his environment reinforces this? Wouldn't it be more surprising if he didn't?

A different psychologist, Kenneth Zucker, PhD, who headed a Toronto clinic for gender identity disorders until 2016, could have told Olson that this was exactly what she could expect would happen. It wasn't about children knowing who they are. If parents and others treated the child as if she or he had swapped sex, the child's gender identity disorder was more likely to persist. Zucker would know. As one of the most respected clinicians and researchers in the field, he'd headed the group that wrote the diagnostic criteria for "gender dysphoria" in DSM-5. The DSM is the "bible" used by mental health professionals throughout the United States to diagnose mental illness. In previous editions, "gender dysphoria" had been called "gender identity disorder," but the name was changed to reduce the stigma that the word "disorder" conveyed. Since it was something that required treatment, whatever it was named, there was no question that it was a disorder. The name change might have seemed a minor issue back then and in line with what trans activists were demanding—the de-pathologizing of their "identities." The DSM authors could not have predicted how major a simple change of wording would turn out to be.

Social transitioning isn't benign. In itself, it's a profound psychosocial treatment. Alleviating the temporary distress a child feels by going along with the child's mistaken perceptions might solve a short-term problem. But it potentially creates a long-term one.

Unlike the children who weren't socially transitioned and who eventually became comfortable with their birth sex, the majority of the "affirmed" kids had no reason to question the notion that they were born in the wrong bodies. Their families became invested in ensuring the kids were treated in every way as if they had magically become the other sex. Family members often became trans activists. So, even if little Johnny wanted to stop pretending he was Jill, how difficult might that be for him? Mom and Dad have been advocating for him to be treated like a girl, yelling, "*Trans rights are human rights,*" at every opportunity. How does he tell them: "*Mom, Dad, I want to go back to being a boy.*"

It would be beyond inconvenient for the entire family. For some, like little Jaron Bloshinsky, even if he'd wanted to, it would have been virtually impossible.

Jaron Bloshinsky, aka Jazz Jennings, was the star of the reality TV show *I Am Jazz*, which promoted the idea that children could change sex and Jaron/Jazz had done it. He became a star by becoming an imitation of a girl.

We don't know whether he would have embraced his birth sex after going through puberty or at some point in adulthood, as almost all young gender-confused kids do, had he not became the poster child for social transition. Jaron never got to experience anything like a normal adolescence. His puberty was blocked. His body's and brain's potential were frozen forever in their prepubescent state, while cameras rolled.

Even the surgery to invert his penis into a neo-vagina was a TV event. The show kept going on and on, despite the horrible complications he suffered due to that surgery.

And if you switched the channel to a different reality show, *Keeping Up With the Kardashians*, you'd see Olympian Bruce Jenner metamorphose into the "transwoman" Caitlyn Jenner.

Aside from what happened to the people in front of the cameras, you have to wonder how this altered the perceptions of the people watching. How much responsibility do these reality TV shows have for driving acceptance of medical and surgical trans interventions, particularly when it comes to children? Most who watched these shows were probably persuaded that trans was the new gay, and that supporting "gender-affirming" care was something akin to an extension of supporting gay rights. It appears to have been one of countless ways that the public was primed to embrace the idea that "trans children" have "identities" that differ from what their bodies say they are—and to welcome research, however dubious, that seemed to prove it.

Kristina Olson won a MacArthur Genius Award for the research that purported to confirm that children's "true identities" could diverge from their physical ones. Meanwhile, two years prior, for his failure to go along with the affirm-all-kids approach that had become the vogue, Kenneth Zucker was fired from his position heading the Toronto gender clinic. Trans activists applauded his ousting. They claimed that Zucker, by helping children explore the reasons behind why they felt gender distress, was engaging in "conversion therapy."

Actual conversion therapy is a brutal and long-discredited behavioral modification scheme that often included electric shock and other horrendous torture-like actions. It was used in earlier decades in an attempt to "cure" homosexuality, which, unlike gender disorders, is a normal lifelong sexuality variation.

For most, identifying as or wishing one were the opposite sex isn't lifelong. Other than in very young children, gender identity distress is most often a symptom of some other psychiatric challenge. Whatever that underlying challenge is, it probably needs treatment.

Yet, transgenderism has been promoted to the public as similar to being gay. It's quickly become conventional wisdom that kids were "born this way," and that to try to figure out what else might be troubling them amounted to an attempt to convert them instead of an attempt to help relieve their distress.

Lawmakers in numerous US states have outlawed ordinary exploratory talk therapy, conflating it with conversion therapy for so-called trans kids. The mere suggestion that other underlying mental health problems could be causing a young person's gender distress—and that solving those problems might also cause the gender problems to abate—has been broadly (and mistakenly) rejected as transphobia.

The same year Olson was awarded her genius grant, Kenneth Zucker wrote a paper explaining why social transition could be seen as "iatrogenic" (injury that's caused by treatment). It puts a child on track for a lifetime of medical and surgical interventions while he or she chases the elusive dream of passing as the opposite sex.

You might be wondering: who decided that blocking a child's puberty was a good idea, and why?

It all began in the Netherlands. Though adults in the country had been able to get cross-sex mimicking surgical and chemical treatments since 1972, a man in a skirt will almost always look like exactly what he is: a man in a skirt. Dutch men who wanted to be viewed as women were regularly disappointed when, despite their efforts to "pass," almost no one was fooled.

Doctors could do nothing for those grown men. But some Dutch psychologists and physicians wondered if they could intervene earlier, before puberty produced the dramatic changes in the body that makes human sex apparent at a glance.

The country's first pediatric gender clinic opened in the city of Utrecht in 1987. Under the direction of the clinic's founder, psychologist Peggy Cohen-Kettenis, PhD, minors were at first offered only counseling. Later, she referred those who continued in gender confusion to endocrinologists in Amsterdam for hormone treatment when they reached the age of sixteen.

One of those endocrinologists, Dr. Henriette Delemarre-van de

Puberty Blockers Come With Profound Risks

Let's pause for a moment and look at the iatrogenic injury that the euphemistically named "gender-affirming care" can do to kids, starting with the drugs prescribed to children between the ages of eight to twelve.

Puberty blockers suppress the gonadotropin-releasing hormone (GnRH) that is normally produced during this time. GnRH prompts the ovaries of girls to begin to produce mature eggs, but if puberty is blocked early on, and a girl goes on to take cross-sex hormones instead of going through natural female puberty, her eggs will almost certainly never mature. She is likely to be sterile.

Breast growth and menstruation are blocked but so is skeletal growth, causing bone weakness and increasing the risk of later osteoporosis.

Because puberty is the time when genitals increase in size, boys on puberty blockers are likely to have only a micro-penis (child-sized) as adults. If the child hasn't yet experienced orgasm before being put on puberty blockers, it's unlikely he ever will. And the gonads, having never gone through male puberty, won't develop sufficiently to produce viable sperm.

The brain also undergoes major changes during puberty. These drugs block that normal brain development, as well, potentially limiting IQ. Among the drugs' side effects are brain swelling and loss of vision—prompting the FDA to require that the drugs carry a "black box" warning.

Though the treatment regimen was sold in part on the promise that blocking puberty is reversible, researchers later determined that that isn't the case, especially not when puberty is blocked for several years.

Waal, had been prescribing a new class of drug, gonadotropin-releasing hormone agonists (GnRHa), to delay precocious puberty (puberty that begins before age eight in girls and before age nine in boys). GnRHa blocks the body from producing the pituitary gland hormones that tell the ovaries in girls and the testes in boys to begin pumping out the sex hormones that surge through a child's body in puberty.

Cohen-Kettenis saw an opportunity to use these new GnRHa drugs to halt puberty altogether, rather than just delay it. That could solve the problem of failing to "pass" as adults.

By the age of sixteen, the children would be prescribed cross-sex hormones. Because they never went through puberty, and the window to do so was now closed, some would never experience orgasm as adults. Some would be forever infertile because the ability to produce mature sperm and eggs was also arrested by the drugs. But the Dutch researchers claimed that this treatment alleviated the children's mental anguish, and that was what mattered most.

But did it actually do what they claimed? Not really.

A study published in 2011, involving seventy adolescents treated between 2000 and 2008, claimed that the treatment improved the children's psychological functioning and relieved their "gender dysphoria."

Viewed as a major success, doctors across the developed world began following the Dutch protocol when presented with gender-confused children: puberty blockers at twelve (in reality, these were often prescribed at much younger ages in clinical practice); cross-sex hormones at sixteen; and genital surgery and mastectomies at eighteen.

Few questioned whether the Dutch protocol had actually cured symptoms of gender distress, despite other researchers being unable to replicate its positive results.

So, Oxford sociologist Michael Biggs, PhD, took a closer look at the Dutch protocol's evidence and found its claims of success were less than they appeared to be.

At the study's onset, the young patients were asked to agree or disagree with a series of statements, with one version for males and an entirely different version for females. Boys who wanted to look like girls were given the male version of the Utrecht Scale prior to getting puberty blockers, with statements such as:

"My life would be meaningless if I would have to live as a boy."

"I feel unhappy because I have a male body."
"I dislike having erections."

The options were "completely agree," "somewhat agree," "neutral," "somewhat disagree," or "completely disagree." If a boy completely agreed with statements like the above, he was considered to have a gender identity disorder.

Right after surgery, instead of giving boys the same series of statements to agree or disagree with, which would have allowed researchers to compare their before and after responses, they gave the boys the opposite sex's version of the Utrecht scale. Granted, the boys no longer had penises, so they would no longer have erections, making questions about how they felt about getting erections moot. But giving them the girls' version made even less sense.

Among the statements the boys were presented with, post-surgery:

"Every time someone treats me like a girl, I feel hurt."
"I hate menstruating because it makes me feel like a girl."
"I wish I had been born as a boy."

A boy who disagreed with these statements was counted as one who longer felt gender distress. Researchers wrote: "gender dysphoria had resolved, psychological functioning had steadily improved, and well-being was comparable to same-age peers."

How could anyone know if that was true?

How could any boy, surgically altered or not, give a coherent response when asked how he felt about getting his period?

The researchers did the same switcheroo with the girls. Their post-surgery responses, like the boys', would be meaningless. Girls have no point of reference on getting erections.

It was impossible to determine anything from their responses.

And one more huge issue was completely ignored. One male patient died as a result of vaginoplasty because puberty blockers had left him with a child-sized penis—too small to perform a penile inversion surgery. Doctor tried substituting a portion of his intestine. It became infected, killing the boy:

As Biggs noted, "A fatality rate exceeding one percent would surely halt any other experimental treatment on healthy teenagers."

It didn't in this case because the researchers omitted his death from their results.

All of this meant the "findings" were fatally flawed and essentially meaningless.

What filtered down to the rest of the world were glowing reports of success. The average physician in clinical practice would assume all was well. The Dutch protocol swept the free world.

If that wasn't bad enough, there was yet another major problem with the protocol. Researchers assumed that anyone with childhood-onset gender disorder who hadn't desisted by twelve years old would have a gender identity disorder for life. If that were true, there would be little to no risk that a child might later desist, embrace his or her birth sex, and regret the procedures. Was this based on sound science?

The answer, as you might have guessed by now, was no.

Alex Byrne, a philosophy professor at MIT, reviewed all the peer-reviewed data on desistance and persistence. He discovered "there is little evidence that childhood-onset gender dysphoria that continues into puberty is 'highly persistent' if not medically treated." Evidence from earlier papers showed the reverse: gender confusion often did resolve later, sometimes as late as young adulthood.

And that meant, prescribing puberty blockers to preteens, on the assumption that their gender disorder was permanent, required making mistakes concerning at least some of the children; probably most of them. Which ones? There's no way to guess.

Once a child is placed on the Dutch protocol conveyor belt, his or her fate is sealed. The child will never get the opportunity to grow up normally.

Children of eight or nine or ten or eleven can't tell you today what they will or won't want from their adult lives, and they can't be taken at their word today if they do. Even if a child were to flat-out say: *"I don't mind being sterile, or having a lower IQ, or weakened bones, or getting no pleasure from sex,"* none of this can be taken as consent. Kids can't appreciate what any of this means.

They're kids.

This should be obvious to anyone who has kids—or, for that matter, anyone who has ever been a kid. Somehow, it's not.

It's not, despite the fact that mental health professionals have known for ages that some children, especially those who will grow up to be same-sex attracted, go through periods of gender confusion. It doesn't make them the opposite sex. Until the trans craze took hold, those who didn't outgrow this phase were rare. The estimates in 2013, when the DSM-5 was published, on those who still wanted to present themselves as the opposite sex by young adulthood? Two or three females in 100,000; five to fourteen males in 100,000.

After puberty blockers, the next drug in so-called gender-affirming care is a cross-sex hormone. Almost all children who are prescribed puberty blockers go directly onto cross-sex hormones. And these prescriptions are typically taken for life.

A Reuters analysis found that the number of children between age six and age seventeen with new diagnoses of "gender dysphoria" nearly tripled in just four years from about 15,000 in 2017 to more than 42,000 in 2021 for a four-year total of almost 122,000. That doesn't include everyone, just the kids who were seen during those four years by medical providers, were diagnosed with "gender dysphoria," and used insurance as payment. About 14 percent of this group of children were prescribed puberty blockers or cross-sex hormones. Since the numbers grew dramatically each year, it's safe to assume the totals are significantly higher now.

Because these figures only include those who sought medical treatment and used insurance, it's also safe to assume that these figures are undercounts.

A paper titled "National Estimates of Gender-Affirming Surgery in the US," which covered the years 2016 through 2020 and was published by the *Journal of the American Medical Association*, calculated that 3,620 of the patients getting breast surgery (3,215) and genital surgery (405) to better mimic the opposite sex were between the ages of twelve and eighteen. A separate analysis found the numbers rising higher from 2019 to 2023, with at least 5,747 minors getting breast and genital surgeries. Those estimates don't include any of Kaiser Permanente's patients; it doesn't make its data available. Yet Kaiser is the largest health provider on the West Coast, with more than half of California's

Cross-sex female hormones (estrogen): When males are given female hormones to help feminize their appearance, the effects can include lessened and softer body hair; increased tissue around the chest area that may resemble female breasts; body fat redistribution; erectile dysfunction; and thinner, dryer skin.

Estrogen appears to increase risks of both prostate and breast cancer in males. It also appears to increase risks of cardiovascular disease, including stroke and heart attack. Overall life expectancy for males who take estrogen is much shorter than in the male population overall. Males also increase their risk of developing autoimmune disorders such as rheumatoid arthritis and multiple sclerosis.

Some males taking estrogen experience major depression. Cognitive functioning can also be diminished, with cognitive decline evident among males who took estrogen long-term, according to one Dutch study.

Cross-sex male hormones (testosterone): When females are given testosterone to masculinize their appearance, the effects include cessation of menstruation; increased facial hair and body hair; a deepened voice; redistributed body fat; an enlarged clitoris; and often, male pattern baldness. The side effects can be significant, and some are permanent, including extreme vaginal atrophy and dryness. Many also complain of constant pain. One study found that 94 percent of young women taking testosterone had pelvic floor dysfunction that caused problems such as incontinence and bedwetting, with more than half experiencing loss of sexual function. Testosterone in females also doubles to quadruples the risk of cardiovascular disease and heart attack, according to one paper. And leaked documents from the World Professional

Association for Transgender Health (WPATH) suggest an increase in liver cancer risk.

That's not even all of it. Testosterone has profound effects on mood and emotions. Helena Kerschner, who took testosterone for several years when she mistakenly believed she was transgender, testified to the Florida Board of Medicine about what the synthetic hormone did to her mental health: "I began experiencing uncontrollable episodes of rage and paranoia where I was a danger to myself and others. I also became more suicidal and self-harming due to this. I was hospitalized twice." Once she stopped taking the drug, her symptoms disappeared.

health-care market, close to half in Oregon, and more than a third in Washington state. It was also the provider for most of the families with gender-confused kids that you'll meet in subsequent chapters. So, the figures above must also be considered significant undercounts.

One reason several experts mentioned for why activists are eager to assert that "trans children know who they are" is that it props up the claims of cross-dressing adults who claim they were "born this way," especially heterosexual adult males with transvestic fetishism or autogynephilia.

"In order to legitimize trans adults, you have to have trans children," says psychotherapist Grace Ellison*.

The existence of "trans" kids gives credence to the middle-aged fetishist when he claims he's always been a female trapped in a male body. The more gender-confused children there are, the more normalized this entirely different disorder that afflicts heterosexual male adults becomes.

You'll read much more about transvestic fetishism/autogynephilia and how it helps drive trans activism in subsequent chapters. For now, what's important to know is that experts in psychiatric sexual conditions believe that most of the adult males who claim trans identities have such fetish-like disorders; they get sexually aroused from either the clothing or imagining themselves to be female or both.

Studies have found that those with autism are six times more likely to claim a transgender identify than those not on the spectrum. That doesn't mean people with autism are more prone to being transgender. More likely, this is tied into how autism can lead kids to become hyper-focused on whatever fires up their enthusiasm. And gender ideology has proved an appealing fixation for young autistic minds. People with autism are also prone to black-and-white thinking. Say, a boy finds that he really enjoys sewing. But sewing is stereotypically considered a female activity. If he has autism, engaging in his favorite pastime might lead him to conclude that this makes him a girl.

But it's not just those with autism who latch onto the trans trend and don't let go. The underlying condition of young people who become convinced they're a different gender might be attention-deficit/hyperactivity disorder (ADHD), sexual trauma, obsessive-compulsive disorder (OCD), post-traumatic stress disorder (PTSD), depression, anxiety, borderline and other cluster B personality disorders (narcissistic, histrionic, and antisocial), or any combination. And that's before considering all the gay, lesbian, and bisexual kids harboring shame about their attraction to others of the same sex. They're especially vulnerable to believing the false promise that "transitioning" will resolve all that by magically turning them into the opposite sex—and therefore, straight.

Stephanie Winn is a licensed marriage and family therapist, and associate producer of *No Way Back,* a documentary about six young people who once believed they were trans but no longer do. Winn has stopped working with minors altogether. That's true of several of the mental health professionals I've interviewed for this book. Their dilemma: they risk losing their licenses if they do exploratory therapy with a kid who self-diagnoses as trans, but the alternative—simply affirming the kid's self-diagnosis—would be unethical.

"Therapists cannot feel the freedom to explore all the various reasons that someone might claim some kind of gender identity," says Winn. "And if we can't explore those reasons we can't get to the root cause of the distress. We can't find out if there's an easier way of treating it."

Winn doesn't believe in the myth of trans children who "know who they are." But, she admits, she once did. She had been the most progressive therapist in a large Portland, Oregon, practice, where she counseled a number of trans-identifying people. When her company held a training in 2017 about how to treat gender-confused kids, she didn't challenge the new mainstream approach she was taught: that a therapist should never question what's behind someone's claim of having been born in the wrong body. When it came to gender, the "customer" was always right, so to speak. Even if kids had other mental health problems, the trainers explained, transitioning was the whole solution. The prevailing theory was that gender distress led to all those other mental health problems that these children had: ADHD, OCD, self-harm, eating disorders, borderline and other personality disorders. Affirm the new identity, the training explained, and all the other mental health problems would go away, too.

Yet, that didn't quite fit what Winn was seeing in her own clients. "It always felt like there was an elephant in the room that we couldn't talk about. Like, what made them think that they were trans, what made them decide to get these surgeries?" she says.

And all those underlying conditions that were supposed to go away once people changed identity? Affirmation wasn't fixing those. Post-affirmation, the same conditions were present in the gender-confused young people she was seeing. Some seemed worse.

In the back of her mind, Winn wondered: was it possible that hormones and surgeries might actually be exacerbating her therapy clients' preexisting problems?

In 2020, Stephanie Winn decided to open her own private practice. Her timing wasn't great. The Covid-19 pandemic was about to shut everything down. But it did give her the breathing space to explore issues that had been stirring in the background, ones she hadn't fully focused on previously.

A friend sent her a link to a *DarkHorse* podcast hosted by husband and wife evolutionary biologists Bret Weinstein and Heather Heying. The hosts offered different takes on topics in the news, which she found persuasive, so she kept listening. Then, on one episode, the hosts discussed an upcoming *60 Minutes* episode that was going to focus on detransitioners.

Detransitioners were people who had once believed they were transgender, only to realize it was all a mistake. They were reverting to identifying as their original sex. But activists were applying pressure, hoping to get CBS to cancel the episode. And CBS was considering doing so. (the segment did eventually air, about two months after *DarkHorse* covered it).

"The reason detransitioners are forbidden and that there would be pressure put on *60 Minutes* is that the strongest argument for a go-slow approach—let us leave children to develop as they will and not leap to conclusions," Weinstein pointed out in the episode, "is that not only does dysphoria so regularly clear up on its own, but that many people who do transition decide later it didn't solve the issue that they were hoping it would solve and decide to transition back. At which point you can't fully transition back, right?"

It was the first Winn had heard of detransitioners. If this new (to her) information was accurate, then almost nothing she'd been led to believe about the need to "affirm" a trans identity and set kids on a course of irreversible medical and surgical procedures could be trusted. The existence of detransitioners changed everything.

Winn has since become one of the most visible and vocal advocates for detransitioners among mental health professionals. While legal and ethical roadblocks make it impossible for her to counsel gender-confused children, she works with their parents, helping them to navigate a world where the entire system is stacked against them. Teachers, counselors, friends, and family members typically buy into the "trans children know who they are" nonsense.

Kids' new "identities" are not just affirmed but applauded in schools in progressive cities like Portland.

And because any exploratory talk therapy at all has been redefined as conversion therapy, there are no therapists left to treat the kids, themselves, for their underlying problems.

"I'm worried about where we're going to be twenty years from now when all of these kids . . . I mean, I think it's going to be tragic," says Winn. "I think there are going to be a lot of people who feel like they're in this in-between land where they know that they are either fundamentally male or female, but they also know that they don't quite look or sound or come across either way. And they'll feel injured physically and psychologically."

That's clearly how Carol feels, one of the many "detransitioners" I've spoken with. She talked of a honeymoon period after "transition" that lasted a few years, when everything seemed wonderful. She'd believed that masquerading as the opposite sex would solve all her concerns, and convinced herself that she was actually meant to be the opposite sex . . . until everything came crashing down.

If you'd asked Carol in 2017, two years after she started injecting testosterone, how everything was going, she would have told you it was great. Fantastic.

Gone, when she studied the person in the mirror, was the image she'd imagined her homophobic mother saw each time she looked at Carol: a woman born wrong, a butch lesbian. Carol had grown a full beard and now looked like a man. Granted, at five-foot-five, she was not the tallest of men, but "Most people will not question a beard."

Everything in life seemed to improve—at least from Carol's perspective.

Her wife had a different view. "She honestly considered maybe I had a brain tumor."

Carol's behavior had become erratic. She'd become more impulsive, making decisions that were way out of character for her. "My mental health was just deteriorating," says Carol. "I felt like it was better. But everybody else around me, and my wife included, was like, this is getting worse."

Carol didn't want to go into specifics about how testosterone affected her behavior, but therapist Stephanie Winn says that although women who take testosterone might find it relieves anxiety and depression, it can also make them more aggressive and angry, cause mood swings, and even bring on psychosis.

On the surface, Carol had had a good thing going before getting swept up in the trans craze. She'd married her first love. They'd recently adopted a son.

Still, Carol couldn't escape the feelings that had been ingrained in her during her teen years: if a woman gravitated toward men's styles, and was attracted to other women, something about her must be broken. So, the trans thing made sense to her. It looked like the fix. The promise, however false, was that she could escape womanhood entirely. She could become Carl*, and in doing so, she could make the wrongness right.

As Carl, she finished college and got a job at a psychiatric hospital for kids, ages twelve through seventeen, acting as a sort of peer mentor.

But one thing jumped out at her immediately after she began working there: more than half the teen female patients identified as trans.

That couldn't be right. Those numbers were statistically impossible. She might not yet have been ready to question her own transition, but how could all these girls be calling themselves boys?

"And then I had a moment where there was a young fourteen-year-old girl there who I could see is probably going to grow up to be a butch lesbian," recalls Carol. "She was very masculine, very tomboy. You could tell she liked the girls but was struggling with that. And I just really felt a compassion and a kinship for her because I understand how that is. And I really wanted, I realized, to tell her that it was okay."

But, of course, "Carl" couldn't say anything like that. As far as the youngster knew, Carol was just some middle-aged dude with a beard. How could "he" begin to understand the sexual identity crisis tormenting a teenage girl?

Though Carol couldn't do much for the teen, the teen helped her, forcing her to look honestly at herself and to feel compassion for herself for probably the first time in her life.

"I was doing the same thing that I wanted to tell her not to do. And so, it's the kids that made me realize my own childish flawed thinking, I guess."

But by this time, as part of her transition, she'd gotten a double mastectomy. Despite her misgivings, Carol believed she had come too far to turn back.

So, she pushed the thoughts out of her mind and kept on as before. Or tried to.

"Fundamentally, you are living a lie," she says. "And that takes an extreme amount of effort to do, to hide all the time, because you're having to hide your sex."

With the whole family living the lie along with her, the strain became intense.

"My anxiety just kept getting worse and worse and worse and worse and I became housebound for the most part. Me and my wife had split up. I was living alone. And I couldn't leave my room because I was having just constant panic attacks."

Carol's wife, meanwhile, was going through her own crisis because the woman she loved was pretending to be a man. She looked for help in online support forums, but her questions were unwelcome. "She was met with, 'If you're not positive 100 percent of the time, you're a TERF, and you're transphobic, and you need to leave.'"

It was the first time she'd encountered the term TERF, short for trans-exclusionary radical feminist.

"To be a support group, you must be open to dissent and you must be open to an honest conversation," says Carol.

Neither was allowed.

One night, alone in her room, Carol watched stand-up comic Hannah Gadsby on a Netflix special. Gadsby joked, sometimes quite poignantly, about the struggles she'd experienced being a butch lesbian. Gadsby could almost be telling Carol's own life story: all the shame; all the stealthy glances of disapproval; all the secret loathing she felt for herself. Carol sat there mesmerized, unable to look away.

"I went, ah, Jesus," says Carol. "I can't do it anymore." And then she sobbed.

She called her wife. She was ready to stop hiding, she said. She was not going to pretend any more—to herself or anyone else. It was hard being a lesbian in a world that didn't want to accept you, but it was what she was. She was a woman. And she was ready to come home.

Her wife cried too. *"Good. Don't do it any more."* Come home.

But when Carol went online to share her journey and hear from others who might be going through something similar, a curious thing happened. Or maybe, not so curious, because it was much like when her wife had gone online to search for support. No one wanted to hear anything trans-related unless it was rainbows-and-unicorns. They certainly didn't want to hear about detransitioning. And they wouldn't tolerate someone who asked questions like, *Just because a woman acted masculine, was that evidence that she was a man?*

"Every single time I stepped in [to an online forum] it wouldn't take but a couple days before I was banned for being transphobic."

She eventually found the connections she craved in a detransition subreddit community. Everyone there had once identified as trans and was now at some stage of detransitioning or considering it. It was a place to tell her story and to hear the stories of others, some painfully similar to her own. People came to ask questions, to say what they couldn't say elsewhere, to lend each other support.

But trans activists weren't happy that a detrans forum existed (which, as of May 2024, had more than 53,000 members).

"They've been what they call 'raided' several times. And one time, they almost lost their account," says Carol. "A raid is when a whole bunch of people on Reddit come in and report a thread or report an account as being against the rules."

Bigotry and hate speech aren't permitted on Reddit; presumably, the detrans group was being reported for hosting both. "Those huge amounts of reports—because it's mostly algorithm stuff—it'll close the account down until Reddit's people can look at it. That's what they would do just to get it shut down all the time."

Carol insists that she saw nothing that would qualify as hate speech on the subreddit. "People were just saying, 'I think this belief system hurt me and I'm mad about it.'"

Carol, too, feels angry, particularly at the professionals who should have protected vulnerable people from making dangerous choices instead of eagerly facilitating them.

"It really boggles my mind that the mental health community has gotten behind this without question," she says.

She's connecting again with in-person lesbian communities and trying to get other detrans lesbians to join the groups. "I think you need it, but it's super hard to find. When I transitioned, there was a lesbian group in my town. When I detransitioned, I couldn't find anything for lesbians. I don't know where they went. There's nothing. It's all trans. It's all trans, and my city is not a big city."

Countless such stories of people who mistakenly believed they could escape same-sex attraction by becoming the opposite sex have led experts like Kenneth Zucker to call "gender affirmation" the true gay conversion therapy. Societal pressure, combined with legally required affirmation by therapists, is converting gay, bi, and lesbian young people to believing they're trans. By the time they realize what they've done, their previously healthy young bodies are irrevocably damaged.

And there's a twist to the story of Kristina Olson's genius-award winning research. Remember her finding that the mental health of affirmed socially transitioned children was essentially the same as that of children who were content with their sex?

It was wrong. She based it on a flawed statistical analysis.

Two other researchers reanalyzed Olson's data with her permission, and found significant errors and omissions. It turns out, when analyzed by more typical, rigorous methods, Olson's data showed that socially transitioned children had significantly *higher* rates of depression and anxiety, and lower levels of self-esteem. Affirming their fantasies didn't lead to better mental health after all.

Yet, you won't find any articles in major media about Olson's faulty data analysis. And the researchers who discovered the issue aren't getting any genius awards. Olson's research has been written of glowingly in numerous prestigious consumer media outlets, which would lead their liberal and moderate readers to conclude that social transition is the right way to go. And Olson's flawed paper has been cited by other research papers, as of June 2024, a total of 1,132 times.

As far as the vast majority of people know, the science is settled on socially transitioning young children, and the results are positive.

None of this is accurate.

If adults can be persuaded, if they can abandon their lifelong understanding that there are two sexes, you're always going to be the sex you were born, and it won't make you happier to pretend otherwise, imagine how easy it would be to convince children. Well, actually, you don't have to imagine. Just read on.

Chapter 2

Consent to This "Care" ... or Else

"I will follow that system of regimen which, according to my ability and judgment, I consider for the benefit of my patients, and abstain from whatever is deleterious and mischievous."

—Hippocratic Oath

"Would you rather have a live daughter or a dead son?"

Countless parents have heard some version of this heart-wrenching question in gender clinics across the United States. Jamie Reed, a former case manager for the Washington University Pediatric Transgender Center in St. Louis, Missouri, admits employing some version of this language on too many occasions in attempts to pressure parents into consenting to experimental treatments on their children.

She believed in those treatments at the time. She believed that what the clinic was doing would ultimately save children's lives. But when Jamie eventually realized that the doctors she worked for were harming, rather than helping, confused kids, she exposed the clinic's dangerous practices. You'll read more about Jamie later.

For now, try to imagine yourself in the place of a mom or dad hearing those words. If you're a parent yourself, you know: you'll do anything to keep your child safe. It doesn't matter whether we're talking about an infant or a full-grown adult. That's your baby. No one gets to hurt your baby. Most of us would step in front of any bullet, whether literal or metaphorical, whizzing toward our kids.

But when the danger is coming from inside a child's own mind—what do you do? Doctors you trust tell you there's no way to completely shield the kid from harm. You must choose between the horrifying—a drastic treatment regime that will alter your child's body forever—and the unthinkable.

Would you rather have a live son or a dead daughter?

How many parents have signed the paperwork, their hearts sinking, telling themselves as they do, *At least she'll still be alive . . . At least now he won't kill himself.*

But have you ever wondered what's behind that warning that's repeated so often to parents? It's unfortunately true that kids who identify as the opposite (or neither) sex attempt or contemplate suicide at astoundingly high rates. But the claim that the only way to keep them safe is to allow them to "transition" is absolutely false.

I know a number of people who have children, grandchildren, nieces, and nephews who have claimed to be transgender. Every one of these family members is politically liberal or moderate. Every one of them probably believes or at one time believed that there was solid scientific evidence to show that when parents don't permit a child to "transition," the child is likely to commit suicide.

But no. There is no such evidence.

Let me repeat: there is exactly zero scientific evidence that you will save your child from suicide by "affirming" that the child is a different sex, or by agreeing to drug-induced or surgical body modifications. There is more evidence that "transitioning" pushes those who go through it *toward* suicide and self-harm than *away* from it.

The trans suicide claims initially sprang primarily from a survey published in 2014 by the Williams Institute at UCLA which recruited respondents via social media.

Called "Suicide Attempts among Transgender and Gender Non-Conforming Adults," it has been used as the basis for the dire warning to parents in gender clinics across the country since it was published. And yet, it never said that "transitioning" kept people from attempting suicide.

It couldn't have done that. It never asked whether the trans-identifying people who claimed to have attempted suicide did so before or after their "transition." So, there is no way to know from the survey whether those who say they attempted suicide were prompted to do so because they were thwarted in attempts to identify as the opposite sex or because they so regretted their decision to do so that they considering ending their lives.

If the survey couldn't determine what effect "transitioning" had on suicide attempts—and this one couldn't—its results are useless regarding the effects of "gender-affirming care" on suicide risk.

A second UCLA survey, done in 2015, that again recruited respondents via the web, came up with similar results but had similar flaws. It was offered to people who identified as trans. Again, though it asked about thoughts of suicide and suicide attempts, there were no questions related to whether transitioning made respondents more or less suicidal.

None.

So, it would be impossible to claim that social, medical, or surgical "transition" had an effect on the risks. Did it make them more prone to suicide? Less? No effect? Since the survey never asked, it can't provide any answers.

It had other significant flaws, too. One of the first questions it asked was: "Have you completed this survey before?"

That's right. Like so many other internet surveys, it had no means of determining how many times a person might have filled out the questionnaire. We've all seen anonymous internet surveys. Some of us have filled them out. Some of us might have been alerted to a survey by politically active friends who hoped to boost the results in one direction or another. And some of us might have taken such surveys more than once to do just that.

But most of us wouldn't rely on the results of such a survey to tell us anything important.

The risks of self-harm up to and including suicide are very real for kids with mental health problems. And most children who imagine themselves to be trans have significant mental health problems. A large study in Finland found that gender-confused young people were, indeed, at higher risk for suicide than the general population. But it wasn't gender-confusion itself, nor was it the lack of "affirmation" that increased the risk. It was their underlying mental health problems. The study found:

Conclusions: Clinical gender dysphoria does not appear to be predictive of all-cause nor suicide mortality when psychiatric treatment history is accounted for.

Clinical implications: It is of utmost importance to identify and appropriately treat mental disorders in adolescents experiencing gender dysphoria to prevent suicide.

But as we saw in the previous chapter, "appropriately treating mental disorders in adolescents" has been reframed when treating the gender-confused as "conversion therapy." A therapist who attempts to understand and treat the underlying cause of a kid's distress risks losing his or her license.

There is no evidence that any of the interventions that are lumped together under the heading "gender-affirming care" decrease the risk. There *is* evidence that adults who have undergone hormonal and surgical interventions to help them mimic the opposite sex are at greater risk of suicide. One Swedish study found that adults who identified as transgender were nineteen times more likely to kill themselves after genital surgery than the general population.

The evidence we do have in no way supports claims that subjecting children to experimental treatments saves them from self-harm. It also suggests that self-reported claims of self-harm and suicide attempts may be wildly inflated. For example, according to a paper published in 2022 regarding teens referred to the United Kingdom's Tavistock Gender Identity Development Services (GIDS), *"In a sample of 900 adolescents (aged from 13 to 17) admitted to the clinic from 2009 to 2017 and given the Youth Self-Report questionnaire, 44% answered that they sometimes or very often 'deliberately try to hurt or kill myself.'"*

Suicide is always tragic, and among kids, more so. But self-reported suicide attempts rarely translate to actual suicide. There were four suicides between 2010 and 2020 among 15,032 GIDS patients. Only two of those patients had already been seen by the clinic; the other two were still on the waiting list.

As the paper goes on to explain, *"The proportion of individual patients who died by suicide was 0.03%, which is orders of magnitude smaller than the proportion of transgender adolescents who report attempting suicide when surveyed."*

Here, again, there's no evidence that social, medical, or surgical treatment or the lack of it had an effect on suicide, and no support for the extortionist question: *Would you rather have a live son or a dead daughter?*

Children in distress need treatment. If it's the right treatment, it could, indeed, potentially save their lives. But "gender-affirming care" isn't that treatment.

And yet, the claim that it is "life-saving" is repeated so often in the media and elsewhere that it's odd to see the phrase "gender-affirming care" without the words "life-saving" or "medically necessary" attached. Virtually every medical association or organization of consequence in the United States repeats the warning, which boils down to: affirm or else.

The World Professional Association for Transgender Health (WPATH) has positioned itself as the premier global authority on both hormonal and surgical procedures—a position that's been accepted virtually without question by media, medical professionals, the legal system, government agencies, and other medical associations. WPATH promulgates "standards of care" for treating those with gender identity disorders, which are treated as gospel by most of these entities. Here's what it says about itself:

> *The World Professional Association for Transgender Health (WPATH) is an international, multidisciplinary, professional association whose mission is to promote evidence-based care, education, research, **advocacy**, public policy, and respect for transgender health.* [emphasis added]

> *... One of the main functions of WPATH is to promote the highest standards of health care for individuals through the articulation of Standards of Care (SOC) for the Health of Transsexual, Transgender, and Gender Nonconforming People. The SOC are based on the best available science and **expert professional consensus**.* [emphasis added]

Note that it considers its mission to include both the promotion of evidence-based care and advocacy. It's worth questioning how one organization can juggle both missions, as evidence and advocacy will at times be in direct conflict. Note, too, that its standards of care are not based solely on "the best available science" but also on "expert professional consensus." As will soon become apparent, these criteria, too, can wildly conflict when the "experts" are all engaged in the "transitioning" industry.

On the FAQs page of its website, WPATH calls hormonal and surgical treatments that are used to alter bodies so that they better mimic the opposite sex "medically necessary, life-saving gender-affirming care."

The American Psychological Association followed WPATH's lead in claims about such procedures, and states that: *[laws limiting children from getting puberty blockers and cross-sex hormones] "would delay access to potentially life-saving care."*

The Endocrine Society agreed: *"Gender-affirming care can be life saving."*

The American Medical Association, too: *""Gender-affirming care is medically-necessary, evidence-based care."*

The Assistant Secretary for Health within the US Department of Health and Human Services in the Biden administration, Rachel Levine, was fully on board: *"Gender-affirming care for transgender youth is essential and can be life-saving."*

Seattle Children's Hospital went a step further: *" ... withholding [hormonal and surgical gender interventions] is harmful to children and amounts to state-sanctioned medical neglect and emotional abuse."*

The American Academy of Pediatrics concurred: *"There is strong consensus among the most prominent medical organizations worldwide that evidence-based, gender-affirming care for transgender children and adolescents is medically necessary and appropriate. It can even be lifesaving."*

It's true that there is a consensus among the most prominent medical organizations in the United States, at least. You'll see similar statements from more than twenty other US medical organizations, even including the American Association for Geriatric Psychiatry and the American Academy of Dermatology (although you might wonder, as I do, how much research into gender-confused children members of either of those groups have participated in).

But maybe you're thinking that it takes quite some hubris for a mere author with no medical credentials to claim that all these illustrious medical professionals got it wrong.

I'd agree, except that it's not just me saying that. It's what the evidence says. And if you scrutinize that evidence with a skeptical but open mind, it's almost impossible not to come to the same conclusion.

Despite the long list of authorities claiming that children need this "life-saving care" and might die without it, the best available evidence doesn't support these claims.

Not one of them.

A huge medical scandal began brewing in the United Kingdom in 2018 when whistleblowers who worked at the Tavistock Gender Identity Development Services in London complained that children were being rushed into irreversible treatments without adequate assessments. The whistleblowers were also concerned about the exponential increases in the numbers of children referred to GIDS. When the clinic began seeing patients in 1989, fewer than ten children a year were referred for treatment, almost all very young boys. Very few were prescribed any medical treatment. Most simply grew out of their gender confusion.

But by May 2021, GIDS had a waiting list of 4,000, with some kids waiting for up to three years. Now, instead of little boys, most of those lining up for treatment were adolescent girls. Such an increase in any other disorder would have sounded alarm bells. That it was affecting young teen girls, a population that had never been affected by gender disorders before, was astonishing.

Just as in the United States, once they were seen in the clinic, most were fast-tracked onto puberty blockers and cross-sex hormones without adequate exploration into why these kids had suddenly latched onto the idea that they were born in the wrong bodies.

And just like in the United States, trans was being viewed as the new gay. People were eager to show their support for the T that had appeared at the end of LGB. Activists insisted that kids knew who they were and would kill themselves if thwarted in their desire to "transition."

But even one of the leaders of the GIDS service agreed that it was "mad" to put any and all children who complained of gender distress on powerful body-modifying drugs.

That madness lit up British media when a young woman named

Keira Bell, who had been prescribed puberty blockers after a visit to the Tavistock GIDS clinic at age sixteen, been given male hormones a year later, and then had a double mastectomy at twenty, realized she'd made a mistake. True, at sixteen, she was certain she knew who she was, and that was a boy. But her certainty dissolved as she matured. She accepted the fact that she was, always had been, and always would be a female. But by then, she was a female without breasts. And she had other significant medical problems, due to her "treatments," that would be with her for the rest of her life. She sued. In an online post, she explained what prompted her action:

> *The consequences of what happened to me have been profound: possible infertility, loss of my breasts and inability to breastfeed, atrophied genitals, a permanently changed voice, facial hair. When I was seen at the Tavistock clinic, I had so many issues that it was comforting to think I really had only one that needed solving: I was a male in a female body. But it was the job of the professionals to consider all my co-morbidities, not just to affirm my naïve hope that everything could be solved with hormones and surgery.*

Keira's story is similar to those of others you'll meet in this book, young people who firmly believed that "transitioning" was the answer to all their problems. Like Keira, when they woke up to reality, often years later, it was too late. Their bodies were maimed. And the medical professionals they'd trusted to fix their problems were the ones who had maimed them.

Between the whistleblower accounts and Bell's, it became clear that GIDS doctors didn't actually understand the consequences of what they were doing. What might be the long-term effects of the procedures they were rubber-stamping, and were those procedures actually making life better for GIDS's patients? No one knew.

Puberty blockers had never been adequately studied in the gender-confused. The drugs weren't even approved for that use. All such prescriptions were off-label. Of the studies that had been done, some were poor quality, others had methodological flaws, and others claimed to find evidence that just wasn't there.

This wasn't what trans activists were saying, of course. According to them, the "science was settled," the treatments were "medically necessary" and "life-saving," and anyone who said differently had ulterior motives.

But unlike in the United States, the United Kingdom's health-care system, the National Health Service (NHS), is government-run. The NHS responded to concerns about GIDS's practices by commissioning systematic reviews of all relevant research and other evidence to determine the bottom line on these treatments.

Pediatrician Hilary Cass was tapped to chair the group and researchers from the University of York assisted with the systematic reviews. These were analyses that evaluated every piece of relevant peer-reviewed literature published to date, to determine what the studies could tell them about social transition, puberty blockers, and cross-sex hormones.

The 388-page Cass Review report came out in April 2024.

Did the evidence say that these treatments were safe?

Did it say they were beneficial?

Did it say they were medically necessary?

The answers, respectively, were no, no, and no.

The Cass Review essentially refuted every claim that all the US medical associations and trans-promoting experts had been making about the benefits of so-called gender-affirming care.

It found no good evidence that social transition was a net positive for children. Like earlier researchers had, the review determined that those children who socially transition (adopting cross-sex names, pronouns, and dress) were more likely to continue on in their gender confusion and to eventually take drugs to stop puberty and mimic the opposite sex.

The review found no evidence that puberty blockers aided in dispelling "gender dysphoria" in children. Nor did blockers increase children's satisfaction with their bodies. The NHS had actually run an early intervention study of the drugs in 2015 to 2016 and preliminary results at that time already showed "a lack of any positive measurable outcomes." But the study results weren't published until 2020. In the meantime, GIDS had kept prescribing the drugs.

As for giving young people cross-sex hormones. "No conclusions can be drawn about the effect on gender dysphoria, body satisfaction, psychosocial health, cognitive development, or fertility." In other words, despite some doctors handing them out like candy, beyond the obvious ways the drugs modified the appearance and functioning of young bodies in the short term, no one had a clue how these experimental treatments were affecting kids' mental health. And no one knew what the long-term physical consequences might be.

The science was anything but settled.

In an interview with BBC, Cass made that point: "I certainly wouldn't want to embark on a treatment where somebody couldn't tell me with any accuracy what percentage chance there was of it being successful, and what the possibilities were of harms or side effects."

In response to the Cass Review, the Endocrine Society had this to say: *"We stand firm in our support of gender-affirming care. Transgender and gender-diverse people deserve access to needed and often life-saving medical care."*

The American Academy of Pediatrics didn't directly address the Cass Report but published a statement that included these two sentences: *"The AAP's gender-affirming care policy, like all our standing guidance, is grounded in evidence and science. Pediatricians understand the complexities of gender-affirming care and they know how to counsel families."*

WPATH came out with guns blazing. *"In contrast to what the Cass Review recommends, WPATH and USPATH firmly stand by the Standards of Care for the Health of Transgender and Gender Diverse People – version 8, which was published in 2022—and based on far more systematic review that the Cass Review—in collaboration with The School of Evidence-based Practice Center at Johns Hopkins University and considers that the (research and consensus-based) evidence is such to recommend that providing medical treatment including puberty-blocking medication and hormone therapy is helpful and often life-saving for young TGD people, while withholding such treatment may lead to increased gender dysphoria and adversely affect psychological functioning."*

Unless you'd read the entire 260 pages of the WPATH Standards of Care, version 8, you would have no idea that it had already directly contradicted its own rebuttal to Cass, with the following statement: *"Despite the slowly growing body of evidence supporting the effectiveness of early medical intervention, the number of studies is still low, and there are few outcome studies that follow youth into adulthood. Therefore, **a systematic review regarding outcomes of treatment in adolescents is not possible.**"* [emphasis added]

If a systematic review of treatment outcomes was determined not to be possible by WPATH, how could it credibly claim that its standards of care for adolescents were "based on far more systematic review" than the Cass Review"?

And yet, it did.

But does that mean Cass was right and WPATH was wrong? Unless you were an expert, how would you know which position to trust?

As it turns out, the United Kingdom wasn't the first and only country to review the evidence on "transitioning" children and to find it lacking. Several other countries had already come to many of the same conclusions as the Cass team and had been putting the brakes on these experimental treatments after realizing that there was no good evidence that they were actually helping kids.

In Finland, an analysis of the effectiveness and safety of giving cross-sex hormones to minors found that the treatment didn't appear to improve their mental health. And since the whole reason for these extreme alterations to the bodies of young people was to alleviate gender-related mental health problems, Finland decided to pull back on so-called gender-affirming care for minors.

Finland's health authority put out a statement concerning gender treatments that "no decisions should be made that can permanently alter a still-maturing minor's mental and physical development."

Swedish authorities, too, had become alarmed. Sweden's health-care policy had been extremely supportive of children undergoing medical gender interventions, and under pressure from trans activists, the country had been considering lowering the minimum age for gender-related genital surgeries from eighteen to fifteen, and allowing children as young as twelve to officially change their sex on their legal records. That was before the country's Board of Health and Welfare reported a 1,500 percent increase in the number of teen girls claiming trans identities between the years 2008 and 2018. Journalists began sounding the alarm about regret among those who had "transitioned" medically and surgically. As the *Guardian* reported in 2020, after a systematic review, "the Swedish Agency for Health Technology Assessment . . . reported that there was very little research either into the reason for the increase or the risks or benefits of hormone treatment and surgery."

Just as in the United States and the United Kingdom, the trans bullet train seemed to be barreling down the tracks with no lights, no brakes, and no clear idea of where it was going.

After reviewing the evidence, the Swedish pediatric gender clinic at the Karolinska Institute, which had been responsible for treating many of these newly gender-confused adolescents, acknowledged the findings and added that the treatments "are potentially fraught with extensive and irreversible adverse consequences such as cardiovascular disease, osteoporosis, infertility, increased cancer risk, and thrombosis."

Sweden's Board of Health declared the risks outweighed the benefits. While not officially banning the drugs, puberty blockers and cross-sex hormones can no longer be prescribed to gender-confused children in the country except under strict controls as part of scientific studies.

France took note of Sweden's findings and urged "great medical caution." Pointing to the increasing numbers of young people who belatedly realized that their gender-confusion was just that, not a new identity, and subsequently detransitioned, the country urged psychological rather than irreversible physical treatments for minors.

In its own systematic review, Norway's Healthcare Investigation Board came to much the same conclusions as Sweden and the United Kingdom, calling gender treatments on minors experimental, and decrying the lack of evidence that these extreme experiments were either safe or effective in treating young people's mental distress.

Given that all these countries were systematically reviewing all available relevant peer-reviewed evidence and coming to almost identical conclusions, you might find it odd that WPATH differed so greatly in its conclusions about how to treat adolescents.

Again, after claiming systematic reviews of evidence in adolescents wasn't possible, WPATH claimed in its rebuttal:

- Its standards of care document (SOC 8) published in 2022 was based on far more systematic reviews than the Cass Review;
- WPATH collaborated with the School of Evidence-based Practice Center at Johns Hopkins University;
- Its research and consensus-based evidence is sufficient to recommend puberty-blocking medication and hormone therapy as both helpful and often life-saving.

What was going on?

Emails from Johns Hopkins that were submitted as evidence in a court case challenging restrictions on transitioning minors show that Johns Hopkins conducted "dozens" of systematic reviews for WPATH. But it "found little to no evidence about children and adolescents."

Yet, the Johns Hopkins researchers were restricted from publishing all but two of those dozens of reviews because of the university's contract with WPATH.

Documents submitted as evidence in yet another court case explain why. Johns Hopkins was required to first get final approval from a SOC 8 leader and "at least one member of the transgender community." WPATH demanded that nothing be published that might "negatively affect the provision of transgender healthcare in the broadest sense."

In other words, if the evidence was at odds with the advocacy, the evidence had to be buried.

It's still unclear what happened to the "dozens" of other systematic reviews the Johns Hopkins team said it completed.

And it wasn't just WPATH pressuring Johns Hopkins. After the organization had a draft of its SOC 8, both the American Academy of Pediatrics (AAP) and the Assistant Secretary for Health within the US Department of Health and Human Services, Rachel Levine, applied their own pressure to WPATH.

Both Levine and the AAP wanted WPATH to remove all minimum age recommendations for treatment from its standards of care document.

According to an expert report from the noted psychologist and sex researcher James M. Cantor, PhD, concerning evidence that is, as of the date of this writing, still under seal in an ongoing case, the American Academy of Pediatrics "issued an ultimatum to WPATH: Should WPATH not delete the age minimums, AAP would not only withhold endorsement of SOC-8, but would publicly oppose the document."

According to that same expert report, Levine, who was born male and began identifying as a "transwoman" in 2011, worried that including any minimum ages might hamper access to the "care" they were all promoting.

In its draft standards of care, WPATH had already, with zero medical justification, reduced the minimum ages from its previous recommendations: approving cross-sex hormones at the age of fourteen (down from sixteen); breast removal at age fifteen (down from sixteen); and both hysterectomies and genital surgeries (other than phalloplasty) at age seventeen. Now, all minimum ages were simply ... gone. Everything was to be left to the discretion of doctors and their underage patients.

This wasn't evidence-based medicine. There was no evidence to support any of this. And where evidence conflicted with advocacy, it was suppressed. This didn't even qualify as "expert professional consensus," despite purported experts being in accord about how to manipulate the document, because the opinions of experts who might disagree were dismissed.

The "standards" for experimental treatments on kids were too often created from vapor, informed by the interests of leading members of WPATH, transgender activists, the American Academy of Pediatrics, and a trans-identifying male in a prominent position within the federal government.

"Gender-affirming care" is such an innocuous phrase—bland and yet somehow soothing. So, before moving on, it's time to become familiar with some of the surgical "care" that WPATH, at the urging of Rachel Levine and the American Academy of Pediatrics, was willing to rubber stamp for kids of any age as long a surgeon was ready and willing:

Top surgery (double mastectomy): Girls as young as thirteen have undergone this surgery to remove both their breasts. The goal is a flat, masculine-looking chest. Side effects can include loss of nipple sensation, permanent scarring, and uneven nipple placement. One of the more serious complications is nipple loss—in other words, the nipples can fall off.

Phalloplasty: The process of creating a facsimile of a penis for a girl requires several surgeries and other procedures. The new organ is fashioned from a flap of flesh that surgeons slice from either the thigh or the arm of a female patient and then roll into a tube shape. This flesh has to be completely depilated first—meaning that all hair and hair follicles must be removed. This isn't as simple as it might sound. Too often, hair removal is incomplete, even when her skin at first appears denuded. A few hairs can cause massive complications because they will keep on growing. But now, they're on the *in*side of the girl's neo-penis, where surgeons have fashioned a neo-urethra. As hair continues to grow, it causes urethral obstruction. In other words, it blocks the ability to urinate.

Other potential complications include bacterial and fungal infections, and failure of the graft. Yes, after all that, a girl undergoing this surgery could be left with nothing. Just pain and scarring. For some, internal scarring can make it impossible to urinate without a catheter. And, of course, the damage to her arm or thigh in order to remove the flesh for grafting is significant, even when the operation is otherwise considered a success.

None of these complications is uncommon. One phalloplasty surgeon says he tells his patients that the complication rate can be 100 percent.

Vaginoplasty: To create a facsimile of a vagina, surgeons cut away much of a boy's penis, then use the inverted skin of the organ to form the tube of an opening that mimics a vagina. It is a complex surgery lasting four to six hours. And because the boy's body experiences the surgery on the penis as a wound and attempts to heal itself, those who get this surgery must "dilate" with a dildo-like device to keep the new canal open.

Although an oft-repeated claim is that such surgeries are never done on minors, a 2017 paper found that about half the WPATH surgeons surveyed had, indeed, performed vaginoplasties on boys as young as fifteen. In boys who have been on puberty blockers, the penis is often child-size so there isn't enough tissue to create a neo-vaginal tube. Jaron Bloshinsky, aka Jazz Jennings, was given these powerful chemicals starting at the age of eleven, and had significant surgical complications as a result when doctors tried to fashion a new vaginal tube for him. He required two additional surgeries to correct the first failed attempt.

Surgeons have tried to solve the problems of using a child-sized penis by surgically removing a section of a boy's bowel and using it as a substitute for a vaginal tube.

Those who have undergone vaginoplasty often develop fistulas between the new vaginal replica and either the bowel or the urethra. Foul-smelling brownish discharge, which can be due to fistula or infection, is a relatively frequent complaint.

Take a good look at "gender-affirming" surgeries. Remember that lobotomies—which essentially destroyed part of the brain by piercing it with a device similar to an ice pick—were also touted as medically necessary for alleviating mental distress.

The young people who are the prime targets for these surgeries might be clamoring for them, but they can't begin to understand the lifelong ramifications. They're kids.

And once done, there's no turning back.

Chapter 3

The Media and the Message

*"What makes it possible for a totalitarian or any other dictatorship
to rule is that people are not informed; how can you have an opinion
if you are not informed?"*

—Hannah Arendt

A government official pressuring a medical society to change its treatment recommendations for political reasons, and that same society burying medical evidence any time it contradicted its recommendations, should have added up to an enormous medical scandal. And it did . . . if you read or watched conservative-leaning media.

In the mainstream press, there was one article and a brief mention in an op-ed in the *New York Times*; one opinion piece in the *Washington Post*, and beyond that, nothing. I'd be surprised if many of my liberal or moderate friends and acquaintances read any of those pieces, and more surprised if they understood the implications of what they'd read.

But the fact that this story made it into such important left-of-center media was the bigger surprise. Because anything that doesn't support the trans activist position usually isn't covered at all, or is subject to extreme "spin." So people whose information sources are moderate and liberal-leaning media learn almost nothing of the profound risks of transgender ideology.

You can't protect yourself or your family from danger when all the reporting you trust informs you that experimental procedures on young people are "life-saving."

Our mainstream media ignore much of what is most toxic about gender ideology, and when they pay attention, most of the reporting ranges from disingenuous to pro-trans propaganda. It's not just that reporters are taking their lead from the medical organizations, and giving the benefit of the doubt to those recognized authorities. Often, trans activists are controlling the narrative. For example, take a look at these headlines from 2022 to 2024, which simply rephrase press releases sent out by trans advocacy organizations such as GLAAD, the Human Rights Campaign, the Trevor Project, and MAP. These are random samples. There are hundreds like this. All sound the alarm about a wave of anti-LGBTQ legislation using the activist groups' language:

"Record Number of Anti-LGBTQ Bills Were Introduced in 2023": *CNN*

"75 Anti-LGBTQ Bills Have Become Law in 2023": *NBC*

"Over 100 Anti-LGBTQ+ Laws Passed in the Last Five Years": *FiveThirtyEight*

"More Than 275 Bills Targeting LGBTQ Rights Flood State Legislatures": *The Hill*

"These 5 States Are Doing the Most to Target LGBTQ People": *Rolling Stone*

"Wave of Anti-LGBTQ Laws Passed across Country": *CBS*

"'I'm Terrified.' Missouri Lawmakers File Onslaught of Anti-LGBTQ bills for 2024 session": *Kansas City Star*

"House Republicans Are Adding Dozens of Anti-LGBTQ+ Measures to Must-Pass Bills": *19th News*

"'War' on LGBTQ Existence: 8 Ways the Record Onslaught of 650 Bills Targets the Community": *USA Today*

They shout almost the identical message: LGBT rights are under attack around the country. Are they?

The scare headlines about a war on LGBT existence, or a wave of anti-LGBTQ laws, have nothing to do with discrimination in jobs or housing, nothing to do with religion-based discrimination against gays and lesbians, and nothing to do with gay marriage.

The laws and bills reported in these articles have almost nothing to do with gay or lesbian anything. The LGB in the headlines is used to provide cover for the T.

It's all about trans. And the "rights" that trans activists have been demanding and getting aren't related to equality. When granted, these new rights typically reduce or eliminate the rights of others, particularly parents, but also women and children in general.

The laws and proposed laws the headlines complain of fall into a number of categories:

- Restrictions on "gender-affirming care" for minors;
- Bans on teaching transgender ideology as fact in public schools;
- Laws permitting parents to opt their children out of transgender and sexual-orientation lessons in public schools;
- Bans on boys competing against girls in girls' sports;
- Bans on boys sharing bathrooms, locker rooms, and showers with girls in public schools;
- Bans on schools socially "transitioning" kids in schools and keeping that change secret from the children's parents;
- And legal recognition that there are only two sexes, male and female.

The only laws or proposed laws mentioned in any of the articles that would restrict or limit anything LGB-related were those that allowed school opt-outs of gender ideology, which sometimes included sexual-orientation lessons. Otherwise, these were all about holding the line against trans demands.

But by calling these laws "anti-LGBTQ" instead of labeling them correctly as pushback against gender ideology, the media outlets were playing on the emotions of readers.

I have no doubt it works. If I saw a headline about "275 Bills Targeting LGBTQ Rights," didn't read the full article, and didn't know what I do now about the way this ideology is promoted, I'd assume that bigotry and discrimination were being cemented into law.

Curious about who was writing these stories designed to scare readers about a war on LGBT people, I checked LinkedIn for information on the authors of the nine pieces I'd picked at random. Almost all the articles were written by reporters who announced their pronouns, identified themselves as LGBTQ, or were relatively recent college grads.

That last factor matters because, in progressive colleges and universities, queer theory isn't limited to gender studies courses. It's central to the culture. It also colors the curriculum at teachers' colleges, law schools, medical schools, schools of social work . . . and, yes, journalism schools. Medill School of Journalism at Northwestern is one of the top schools of journalism in the country. It also has an endowed chair in sexual and gender minorities journalism. Like academia in general, journalism schools preach the need for graduates to take up the cause in the name of social justice.

Because it was drilled into them at school, not just in their classes but wherever they gathered on campus, younger reporters are more likely to view gender ideology as something it is their duty to defend, rather than just report on. So when major media organizations fill their newsrooms with earnest young social justice warriors, you get pieces like the one that appeared on New Year's Eve 2024 in the *New York Times* under the heading, "Ohio Is about to Make Queer Kids Miserable."

Its youthful self-described "queer" author wrote that Ohio's pending Parents' Bill of Rights legislation was an attempt to create a *"sinister surveillance state that directly targets L.G.B.T.Q. kids for discrimination,"* adding that, *"Should their parents be at all queerphobic, the consequences of state-mandated outing will be dangerous, if not deadly. And even if young queer people manage to covertly endure such a measure, they will be forced by their government to contend with the sort of shame that kills too, albeit more slowly."*

Sounds terrifying, doesn't it?

What does this *"sinister surveillance state"* legislation actually do? Here's a summary:

- Acknowledges that parents have the fundamental right to make decisions regarding their children's upbringing;
- Guarantees parents the right to access their children's education and health records;
- Prohibits school personnel from encouraging children to withhold information about their health from their parents;
- Prohibits sexuality and gender ideology lessons for children between kindergarten and grade three;
- Gives parents the option to review all sex ed materials and opt their

kids out, if they choose;
- Requires that sex ed be age and developmentally appropriate;
- Requires that the school inform parents of any counseling or other health-related services their children get at school;
- Requires that the school notify parents of changes in their children's wellbeing, including identifying as something other than a child's actual sex.

That's it. Much of the above is common sense. And most of the rights granted by the legislation are those that parents *already* have under federal law and the Constitution, though indoctrinated school personnel sometimes act as if parents are so "unsafe" that respecting parental rights poses a threat to children. This line from the *New York Times* piece typifies that attitude: "*the consequences of state-mandated outing will be dangerous, if not deadly.*"

So what exactly is this "queer theory" that's tinged the way our mainstream media report on gender ideology?

Like critical race theory, queer theory is considered an offshoot of postmodernism, an academic school of thought that rejects the idea that humans can grasp objective truth or knowledge. Postmodernism especially rejects authorities who claim to have or teach knowledge. In simple terms, postmodernists view authorities as oppressors.

Queer theory applies these academically brewed concepts of social justice to sex. Eager to "queer" (disrupt) rules governing sexual behavior, it rejects the idea that anything about sex should be considered either normal or deviant. Sex is simply sex. Attempts to categorize or define specific sexual acts and desires as normal or not, any regulation of sexual behavior, and any shaming of people whose sexual tastes are atypical, are forms of oppression. Queer theory adherents also reject the laws of nature that make human sex binary, either male or female. Trans ideology falls under its umbrella.

Although its academic beginnings give it an intellectual gloss, queer theory is, was, and always will be about sex, about doing whatever you want to do sexually and demanding acceptance for it.

In practice, proponents of queer theory are dismissive of, and often ridicule those in one broad category of sexual behavior: heterosexuals who know human sex never changes and are fine with that.

Queer theory is, in a word, absurd. But it's also become a force in society, particularly because it's the lens through which activist journalists view and report anything trans-related.

Americans overwhelmingly support equal rights for those who identify as LGBT. We know this because, for about a decade, the Public Religion Research Institute (PRRI) has polled people across the country every year, asking whether they support or oppose the following:

1. Laws that would protect gay, lesbian, bisexual, and transgender people against discrimination in jobs, public accommodations, and housing.
2. Allowing a small business owner in your state to refuse to provide products or services to gay or lesbian people if doing so would violate their religious beliefs.
3. Allowing gay and lesbian couples to marry legally.

Americans consistently say they support laws that protect the rights related to the first and third questions. They believe everyone should have equal rights when it comes to jobs, public accommodations, or housing. They want gays and lesbians to be free to marry. And they don't believe businesses should be able to use religion to discriminate against gay and lesbian people.

There's a downside to the incessant linkage of the LGB and the TQ, though. Consistently conflating the same-sex attracted with the trans-identifying has gained sympathy for the T group (while the Q part of the abbreviation goes largely unexplained). But as more people reject trans ideology, some might also turn against gays and lesbians.

Some evidence suggests that it might already be happening. The most recent (as of this writing) PRRI survey shows a slight dip in Americans' support for gay rights for the first time since the survey began. Support for gay marriage had risen to an all-time high of 69 percent in 2022. In 2023, it dropped to 67 percent. The percentage of those who were against discrimination in employment, housing, and public accommodations fell from 80 percent in 2022 to 76 percent in 2023. And opposition to allowing small businesses to use religious grounds to discriminate against gays and lesbians fell from 65 percent of Americans to 60 percent.

When media treat propaganda of any sort as objective information, we all lose, even if it isn't evident in the moment. And if you're not yet persuaded that that's what's happening, another writer who's been covering transgender issues, Jesse Singal, discovered a different major media trans-propaganda pattern. In thirty-five articles, bylined by about twenty different writers, published by CNN over about two years, this same sentence appeared, either verbatim or close to it:

> *Gender-affirming care is medically necessary, evidence-based care that uses a multidisciplinary approach to help a person transition from their assigned gender—the one the person was designated at birth—to their affirmed gender—the gender by which one wants to be known.*

It even appeared in an article that announced that the United Kingdom was no longer prescribing puberty blockers because there was "not enough evidence to support the safety or clinical effectiveness." The article went on to repeat the false claim that puberty blockers' effects are reversible. And, it included another obligatory statement that "every major medical association agrees that gender-affirming care is clinically appropriate for children and adults. This includes the American Medical Association, the American Psychiatric Association, and the American Academy of Child & Adolescent Psychiatry."

The line between transgender propaganda and information has been blurred by mainstream media for years, which in large part explains why most who are left of center politically have no clue about the hazards, and believe in the purported benefits. Most left-leaning consumers of mainstream media have internalized the messages that male and female are outmoded concepts; sex occurs on a spectrum; and there are trans children all around us, just waiting for the right moment to "come out"—and when they do, they need monstrous body-altering chemical and surgical interventions, euphemistically called gender-affirming care, to keep them from killing themselves.

None of it is true. But when your media sources, your doctors, your mental health professionals, and everyone you know buys into these claims, you can start believing it, too.

Sometimes, the disinformation is subtle. At other times, it's remarkably clear.

In April 2024, a colleague forwarded an intriguing article to me that had run in the *Sacramento Bee*. The headline read: "A Mom of a Nonbinary Teen Became an Anti-Trans Activist, Fracturing a California Family." The headline suggested that whatever had befallen this family touched by the trans craze, the mom, Beth Bourne, was the villain of the story. I became more intrigued as I read. Her daughter, as a preteen, had begun thinking of herself as a boy. She'd changed her name several times since, and now at age eighteen, wanted to be considered non-binary.

I'd seen this movie before—different characters but essentially the same script.

The first of my friends to have a trans-identifying child in her family was Eva*. Her oldest granddaughter, Natalie*, suddenly decided she wanted to be called Nathan*. Within about six months, her parents agreed to fly her to another state to have her breasts removed—paying out-of-pocket rather than trying to get their insurance to cover it. This "life-saving" care must have seemed so urgently necessary that they just couldn't ask her to wait.

And yet, about a year later, Natalie wasn't calling herself a boy any longer, and she wasn't wearing boy's clothes. She now claimed to be "non-binary." Her favorite outfits were rompers, those cute little ultra-feminine skirted jumpsuits. But Natalie was as hairy as any boy due to the testosterone she'd taken while she identified as Nathan. And she no longer had breasts.

Then, last year, Natalie's cousin Maggie*, twelve at the time, decided she wanted to be called Matthew* and use he/him pronouns. Fortunately, a recent photo of "Matthew" that Eva sent me shows Maggie wearing makeup and a very sexy crop top—about as un-masculine as you can get. Still, Eva isn't sure what will happen next. Natalie's little sister has begun using they/them pronouns.

Eva has only one grandchild out of four, a boy, who isn't identifying as something other than his actual sex.

Then, there's my friend Jodie*. Her first-born, Tabitha*, decided she was a boy, then non-binary, then a boy again. A couple of name changes went with the identity changes. A few years after Tabitha's "transition," Jodie's youngest, Peter*, decided he was a girl. As far as I know, Peter didn't have surgery, which is a relief, because he no longer imagines himself a girl. He, like Natalie, claims to be non-binary, and has chosen Kelly* as his new gender-neutral name. (The term "non-binary" is essentially meaningless, but it allows kids to stay connected to their "queer" communities even if they revert in every other way to their actual sex.)

Most recently, someone in my extended family told me his fifteen-year-old niece is "transitioning." Knowing where it could lead, I begged him to talk his former brother-in-law out of going along with her new name and pronouns. But it was already done.

It was also too late for the niece of the colleague who'd sent me the article. That sixteen-year-old recently had a double mastectomy.

Other than these newest recruits to the child trans cult among my friends and family, the others have already changed identities, names, wardrobes, or pronouns at least once.

These kids do *not* know who they are.

So, when I read in the *SacBee* that Beth Bourne's daughter was on her fourth name, and second trans identity, I figured that the situation might be a little different from what the paper was reporting. I got in touch with Beth to get her side of the story.

Beth Bourne seems so fragile when she speaks of her daughter. I almost expect her at any moment to crumple. It's obvious that she's holding in tremendous pain. Her eighteen-year-old first-born Elisa has cut off all contact with her. It's now more than a year since they've spoken.

For years, Beth yielded on almost everything: pronouns, new name, and a whole new wardrobe purchased from the boys' department. She would not relent on her child's most hazardous requests though: puberty blockers and cross-sex hormones.

Since seeing the relationship with her daughter dissolve, she's made it her mission to alert other parents to dangers she herself knew almost nothing about until it was too late.

Though the article blamed Beth for tearing her family apart, she hopes people will read between the lines and recognize the truth.

That seems unlikely, especially with passages like the following:

"Beth's politics became more extreme."

"But this crusade has taken an increasingly fanatical turn."

"Beth . . . increasingly radicalized."

But as I found when I went through the copious documentation of her daughter's and her journey that Beth shared with me, I discovered she is neither extreme, nor fanatical, nor radical. She's just a mom who got blindsided and tried her best to save her child.

Like so many other parents of gender-confused kids I've interviewed, Beth was a lifelong Democrat. If she knew that the school her kids attended was committed to "social justice," it wouldn't have concerned her. Beth Bourne was unaware of the dark side of what passes for social justice today.

She was surprised when her daughter arrived home from class one day claiming a new sexual identity. Eleven-year-old Elisa declared that she was bisexual. It's impossible to know how many prepubescent kids come home from a "sex ed" class having adopted one of the sexual identity labels they learn about there: bisexual, pansexual, polyamorous, agender, and others. But as has been true for countless other kids, it was Elisa's first stop on the trans train.

Elisa was also coping with her first exposure to sexual trauma. Her best friend in sixth grade had witnessed a sexual assault on another child. She didn't report it, but told Elisa. The incident affected the girls deeply. They were also watching the Netflix series *Thirteen Reasons Why* about a teen who committed suicide. Both girls started to think and talk about killing themselves.

"My daughter just became really withdrawn that whole summer and was on her phone a lot," recalls Beth.

According to several therapists, when a kid is exposed to sexual trauma—even when it happens to someone else and not herself—it can make a girl want to escape womanhood.

As Elisa started seventh grade, her mental health deteriorated. She began cutting herself.

Beth knew something was terribly wrong. She sensed that it might be tied to the sexual assault. The worried mom didn't know it at the time, but the school had been promoting transgender ideology to students. Those lessons coming when they did might have made a weird sort of sense to a twelve-year-old girl: elude your angst by becoming someone else. She began dressing like a boy. She chopped away her long pretty dark blonde hair and wore what was left in a boy's style.

"Her father and stepmother immediately took her to the Sacramento Lavender Library, it's an LGBTQ library, and they took her to Pride Festivals, and they let her check out the book *I Am Jazz* about Jazz Jennings."

Far less willing to embrace Elisa's out-of-nowhere decision to present as a boy, but desperate for her daughter to be well and safe, Beth would eventually agree to almost everything, even a binder to flatter the girl's breasts so she'd appear more masculine. But she was still uneasy with how far her ex seemed willing to go.

Both parents decided to enroll Elisa in an intensive dialectical behavioral therapy (DBT) group where the girl would learn skills that they hoped would help her manage her stress and keep her from further injuring herself. Elisa also began taking an antidepressant to treat what her psychiatrist diagnosed as an anxiety disorder.

But in eighth grade, Elisa's emotional state worsened. Formerly an A student, she began getting Ds and even Fs in all her classes except PE, choir, and Spanish. And she was still cutting herself. One day in school, she sliced into her thigh so deeply, it required stitches.

Sometime in November 2018, in the midst of all this, Elisa wrote letters: one to her father, and another to her mom. She began the one to Beth by saying, "As you undoubtedly know, I am trans. My name is Ian, pronouns he/him." She also wrote that "nothing medical is necessary for many years."

Soon after, the school changed the eighth grader's name to "Ian" on all her records.

You'll see nothing about Elisa's mental health struggles in the *SacBee* article. Instead, this is what the reporter wrote about the above period, using Elisa's most recent name "Lily" and her current "they/them" pronouns:

> *Conflict between parents and their adolescent children is normal, if not expected. But for Lily, the constant fighting and denial of their person-hood went deeper than everyday bickering—they were sharing a roof with a mother who actively, publicly, opposed the person they were becoming.*

"I was ready to come out to everybody because I had been holding it in for a really long time," Lily said. "From my coming out to my moving out, her views that she expressed to me started to get more aggressive and more extreme."

The *SacBee* article made it sound as if Elisa's life magically changed for the better because she imagined herself a boy, and the only aspect of life that wasn't great as a result was her mom's resistance. In truth, at that point, as evidence she emailed to me showed, Beth wasn't resisting much at all. But Elisa was still in a bad state, mentally and emotionally. Two months after officially "coming out"—and more than a year after starting to present as a boy—she carved an unsettling message into her arm with a razor.

Beth has voluminous school, medical, and court documentation that she shared with me, and with other reporters and writers. She would have shared with any writer who was interested. But the *SacBee* reporter either didn't ask or didn't look. Here's what the reporter wrote about this period, from which a reader would gather that it was Beth, not Elisa, who was experiencing a mental breakdown:

As [Elisa] embraced their trans identity, they grew happier. Their father and stepmother affirmed the transition. Beth remained concerned about it, and increasingly radicalized. In so doing, she isolated herself not just from her child, but her community.

Elisa's mental health did, at last, show noticeable improvement once she began ninth grade. Whether due to the coping mechanisms she learned in therapy or the antidepressants or both, as the youngster's emotional turmoil abated, the cutting stopped, and her grades improved dramatically.

But Elisa's assurance, at age thirteen, that "nothing medical is necessary for many years" was no longer operative by the time she turned fourteen.

Her parents took Elisa to see her doctor at Kaiser Permanente, a managed care company, because the girl was having dizzy spells. While there, the doctor overheard Elisa's father call her by male pronouns and offered to change her medical records to reflect that. "And then the pediatrician said, '*You should go to Kaiser's Gender Proud clinic in Oakland*,'" recalls Beth. " '*It's a one-stop shop where you can meet with an endocrinologist.*'"

At this "one-stop shop," which Beth says she is certain are the words the doctor used, the endocrinologist could prescribe the pretty young teen, first, puberty blockers, and then, cross-sex hormones.

The doctor assured the parents the drugs could be safely administered. Elisa's father was open to the idea. Like so many other parents, he apparently believed he could trust a pediatrician's word.

Beth wanted to see the evidence to back that up. She had been researching since Elisa declared herself a boy. In late 2019, there was still very little resistance to the dominant narrative that these powerful chemicals were just fine to give to children.

"My daughter's psychiatrist . . . texted me the article that Jesse Singal wrote from the *Atlantic*," says Beth. "These parents were pushing back on [kids claiming to be trans] and they were finding that their daughters were, you know, were growing out of the identity."

She decided to call the Kaiser endocrinologist to ask about the drugs. "He said, you know, it's an emerging science, but we know that you can successfully put kids on these puberty blockers to 'buy some time,' and then use testosterone or estrogen to help kids, you know, whatever, affirm their gender identity."

He painted the drugs as benign but the term that stuck in Beth's mind was "emerging science."

So, there were no long-term studies?

None.

No one knew what might happen to these children in ten, twenty, thirty years?

Correct. No one knew.

That meant, her daughter would be among the guinea pigs.

She had been acquiescing to so much. But she could not acquiesce to that.

As she drove her daughter across town one day, she explained her decision. "I said, 'I would let you have your breasts amputated before I would let them put you on testosterone or puberty blockers. Because I know if you take your breasts off, you've lost your breasts, you've lost your ability to breastfeed. But if I put you on testosterone, I don't know how that's going to affect your brain development, your bone density, your fertility, because it's never been studied.'"

She offered Elisa a compromise. She would let her go on a type of birth control that would stop her period almost completely.

Meanwhile, she had to explain what was going on to her son, who was almost three years younger than Elisa.

At the end of her junior year in high school, Elisa asked Beth to come with her to speak to her therapist. Beth recalls the visit. "She said, 'Mom, this is going to be hard for you to hear, but [the therapist] knows. I'm going to be living with Dad all summer.'"

Beth had done enough research by now to expect something like this. Dad was fully affirming and she still was resisting. She'd fought when Elisa decided at the tender age of fourteen to legally change her name to Ian. Elisa's birth certificate, passport, all her papers now all said that she was born male. Beth had refused to allow the teen to go on the powerful chemical body modifiers that her ex was willing to endorse. As her daughter got closer to her eighteenth birthday, the age when she would be free to get a prescription for cross-sex hormones without parental consent, Beth worked harder to persuade her that she was and always would be female, no matter what her birth certificate now said.

"But now I realize you almost can't do that, right? If you're in a cult . . . Your parents say there's no such thing, they're not going to believe you, right? And then, you know, the cult says you need to go 'no contact' with that parent."

Beth says that Elisa, her father, and her stepmother were united in the belief that Beth was a transphobe.

"I did get her to go on a trip the end of that summer," says Beth. "We went to Bangkok, and we went to Tokyo together. And it was really fun."

They got back just in time for Elisa's seventeenth birthday. It was a typical celebration with the family around Beth's dining room table. There were cake, balloons, and presents. Beth gave Elisa a special watch she'd bought while they were in Japan. For that moment, they were all happy together.

"And then she walked out of the room on her seventeenth birthday and she never came back."

Beth managed to see Elisa from afar at school choir and theater events, and at her son's volleyball games.

During her senior year of high school, Elisa was still going by "Ian," but Beth noticed a few changes as she watched from a distance. First, Elisa was wearing nail polish. Then, her daughter began dressing in more feminine styles, even on occasion, wearing skirts. She used mascara. And she was dating a boy.

Beth held out hope that Elisa might be in the early stages of desisting.

The mom had already begun a deeper dive into the ideology that had ruptured her family. She was involved in online groups such as Parents With Inconvenient Truths About Trans (PITT) for the parents of gender-confused kids. Through other moms, dads, and relatives, she'd discovered how similar many of their experiences were.

Since then, she's become a regular at school board meetings, pushing back against the extreme indoctrination in the district. She's also hosted a number of events outside the school that expose the falsehoods being treated as fact. Though she does her best to alert parents, the whole city seems ideologically captured. It's almost impossible to break through. But there's no question that she's a mom on a mission, just as other mothers and fathers of gender-confused kids (some now desisted, others still seduced by the cult) make it their mission to sound the alarm, hoping they can save other families from what theirs went through.

And in July 2023, this lifelong Democrat took over the chair position of Moms for Liberty, Yolo County chapter, a parents' rights group, founded by conservatives, which has attracted parents from across the political spectrum whose children have been negatively affected by trans ideology.

Beth would have preferred working with a liberal or moderate group to counter the ideology. But no such liberal or moderate group exists— although other Moms for Liberty members share her moderate political views on other issues. So when Beth gets media attention for her chairing of the local chapter, her political history is rarely mentioned. Instead, she's painted as a rightwing extremist, which signals to liberals and moderates that they can safely ignore her warnings and dismiss her as a crank.

Elisa, meanwhile, apparently switched from identifying as a boy to non-binary sometime in her senior year of high school. She can be seen providing public comments on video at a school board meeting, where she complained that "my mother is a part of this group who is protesting against my rights."

Elisa got riotous applause from the crowd behind her, many of whom held up signs in the pastel rainbow colors associated with trans ideology sporting such slogans as "No Hate In Our Town"; "No More Hate In Davis"; and "Davis Says NO To Transphobia." Elisa was the last of about a dozen speakers, all of whom spoke in favor of the school board's trans policies, and all of whom were encouraged by cheers and applause from the sign wavers and others behind them. Two of the speakers repeated the extravagantly false claim that "trans" children who aren't affirmed have a 50 percent chance of attempting suicide.

By the end of high school, Elisa had changed her name to "Jude." And at some point during her freshman year at college, she changed her name again, now using the female name, "Lily," although she still claims to be non-binary and part of the queer community.

But if you read the *SacBee* article, you'd be assured that first trans, then non-binary, Elisa (aka "Ian"/"Jude"/"Lily") was certain of who she was. Just like every other magical trans child.

This inability to see what's in front of their noses appears to inform so much pro-transgender mainstream media reporting.

There's no war against the LGBTQ community, no war even against that T toward the end—just resistance to something that's happening in plain sight that harms children. There does, however, appear to be a war against non-affirming parents. And as you'll see in the next chapter, their children's bodies are the battleground.

Chapter 4

Today's Lesson: Reject Your Sex

"Now, the kinds of issues and the kinds of lessons that are being pushed are at very, very young ages and often with extremely graphic and sometimes disturbing content."

—Nicole Neily, Parents Defending Education

It's not difficult to see how an adult like Carol, who you met in chapter 1, could be seduced into imagining she's the wrong sex. Trans ideology greets people everywhere, even when it's subtle. It's in the diversity, equity, and inclusion (DEI) training you're required to complete at work. It's in the news you consume. If you're gay, lesbian, or bi, other members of your community have probably already decided to "transition." If you have any kind of social life, whether you get together in person with friends, or it's just you, your smartphone, and your anonymous online social media connections, you can't completely escape exposure to the dogma.

But how does a young child get the idea that he can change sex, i.e., gender, or have no gender at all? Why are first, second, third, fourth, and fifth graders adopting "queered" non-binary and trans identities?

We know that something unprecedented began happening in the second decade of the twenty-first century. The surge in the number of people trying to identify out of their sex, especially among adolescent girls and young women, has been staggering.

As you might recall from earlier in the book, as of January 2022, UCLA's Williams Institute doubled its estimate of the prevalence of kids thirteen to seventeen openly identifying as trans or non-binary nationwide from 7 in 1,000 (0.7 percent) to 14 in 1,000 (1.4 percent). But national figures don't tell the full story. State-by-state estimates showed a wide variance: 0.6 percent of teens in Wyoming were gender-confused compared to 3 percent of teens in New York.

That's a whopping five times greater prevalence in New York than in Wyoming.

A Centers for Disease Control (CDC) survey the following year found that even those estimates were way low. By 2023, 5.5 percent of high school students nationwide either said they were trans or thought they might be. In some hotspots, the numbers are even more striking. The Oregon Department of Education calculates the number of gender-confused kids in its schools at 8 percent. In a survey of high schoolers in one Pittsburgh school district, more than 9 percent claimed a trans or non-binary identity.

Most newly gender-confused teens developed what researcher Lisa Littman, MD, named rapid onset gender dysphoria (ROGD). A better name for the phenomenon might be socially induced gender identity disorder, which adds the how to the what. It's a mental health disorder spread by social contagion.

Social contagions, or mass psychogenic illnesses as they're also known, are not new. Groups of girls in earlier years have developed eating disorders together, and have claimed to have developed Tourette's syndrome, multiple personality disorder, fits, trance states, and fainting episodes together. One mass psychogenic illness occurred in the 1980s to 1990s due to a trend among mental health professionals who believed that their patients had developed amnesia about brutality inflicted on them when they were small children. So these mental health professionals induced suggestible patients to recall "repressed memories" of that buried trauma while under hypnosis or after deep relaxation exercises. Patients began recounting vivid reminiscences of horrifying events that seemed to prove the therapists correct: they had tapped into suppressed memories. The problem was that the "memories" were of trauma that had never actually happened. These therapy patients began falsely accusing relatives and others of committing unspeakable acts—not unlike the Salem witch trials, yet another case of mass psychogenic illness.

In the current mass psychogenic contagion, the major influencers among newly indoctrinated teens tend to be the other teens they hang out with and the websites they visit. The ideology is promoted on Reddit, Discourse, Tumblr, Twitter, YouTube, TikTok, and even in anime cartoons, along with countless other virtual spaces and special interest forums. A kid with a smart phone is a kid who has either been exposed to transgender proselytizing or is about to be. Some experts also mention underage indoctrination via readily available online porn (particularly, for boys, a trans subgenre called sissy hypno porn). All these both allure teens and cement the notion that people can be born with mismatched brains and bodies.

But proliferation on the web fails to explain how and where the contagion is introduced to smaller children.

Who plants that first seed? What's primed so many youngsters who don't yet know what sex is to be susceptible to the notion of altering their identities and bodies? Why would the average child imagine that changing sex is even possible?

This ideology is snowballing and it's drawing in younger and younger children. How?

Just ask Beth Bourne. Before they get their first smart phones, before they discover this thing called TikTok, before they're even allowed to use the home computer unsupervised, there's one outside influence affecting almost all children.

School.

One Portland, Oregon, area mother told me that in her eight-year-old son's second-grade class, where kids are asked to announce their pronouns daily, three children identify as non-binary. That class has only sixteen children.

Three out of sixteen had already rejected their sex by the age of eight?

In a different city, one mom, proud that she had enrolled her child in a school that was "anti-racist, inclusive, and believes in social justice," soon became horrified after the school taught a class on "identity." That lesson persuaded one-quarter of the eleven-year-old girls in her daughter's class that they were boys . . . including her own child.

You know the old horror movie trope: the call is coming from inside the building.

Queer theory has spread, largely by stealth, through K–12 classrooms, disguised as "comprehensive sex education." The activists who write so-called sex ed curriculum materials largely reject the notion of childhood innocence, claiming that preserving innocence limits a child's freedom and forces the child into a "cis-heteronormative" framework. Queer theorists also reject what earlier experts, such as Jean Piaget, determined about children's cognitive development. Instead, according to one influential paper, "developmental theory and its attendant model of Developmentally Appropriate Practice (DAP) can be destructive to some children's imaginative and social capacities when not attuned to their possible queer presents and futures."

While that sentence is ludicrous in its own right, what's happening in progressive school systems is worse than that makes it appear. That's because the queer theorists in charge of creating "comprehensive sex education" (CSE) materials aren't simply making assumptions about potential "queerness" in children just waiting to be discovered. CSE is more a recruitment strategy than actual sex education. It's queer theory for children.

And just like queer theory for adults, it involves denial of biological reality and a commitment to warped notions of social justice.

But it's much worse than the indoctrination exercises aimed at adults. Adults have access to all manner of information and can theoretically, at least, independently research, determine that gender ideology is closer to a religion than it is to science, and dismiss it. A five-, six-, or seven-year-old? That child is a captive audience, with no way to distinguish queer theory fantasy from reality. That child, from the time she or he first enters school, is being molded into a disinformed social justice warrior. The child will be lied to about what sex actually is, and will be actively encouraged to reject his or her own.

All this happens in "sex ed" classrooms, and in less formal settings, in gender ideology groups with names like "Rainbow Club" and "Skittles" sometimes as early as pre-K.

The re-jiggering of sex ed into what amounts to a conversion experience breaks down the boundaries that most parents rely upon to shield their children from sexually explicit concepts and behavior.

A group of influential queer theory–based sexuality education contractors that includes SIECUS, Planned Parenthood, and Advocates for Youth, calling their collaboration the "Future of Sex Education," created a document, "National Sex Education Standards," that outlines what CSE should cover. It's been formally adopted by a few states, while several others and numerous more progressive school districts around the country informally rely on it to inform their sex ed curriculum. The document cautions that sex ed "should avoid cisnormative, heteronormative approaches," disregarding that most children, if left to their own devices, will grow up heterosexual, while a handful will be gay or bisexual. CSE doesn't want to leave kids to their own devices, though. Everything must be "queered," and children must see the queer viewpoint as the correct one.

To give you an idea of how this plays out in practice, the National Sex Education Standards sets study and learning goals for different grades. By the end of second grade, for example, children are expected to be able to:

- Define gender, gender identity, and gender-role stereotypes;
- Discuss the range of ways people express their gender and how gender-role stereotypes may limit behavior;
- Demonstrate ways to treat people of all genders, gender expressions, and gender identities with dignity and respect.

Of what possible benefit is it to a second grader to be taught to believe the false claim that there are multiple genders? What advantage does that second grader gain from discussing how others might express gender confusion? Second graders are too developmentally immature for any kind of sex ed. But this isn't even sex ed. This is gender ideology indoctrination.

The standards for what children must learn by the end of fifth grade are at least as problematic:

- Describe the role hormones play in the physical, social, cognitive, and emotional changes during adolescence and **the potential role of**

hormone blockers on young people who identify as transgender;
[emphasis added]
- Distinguish between sex assigned at birth and gender identity and explain how they may or may not differ;
- Define and explain differences between cisgender, transgender, gender non-binary, gender expansive, and gender identity;
- Explain that gender expression and gender identity exist along a spectrum.

This, again, serves only one purpose: to indoctrinate children into a belief system. Other than the nod to hormones, these lessons have no basis in biology, and no place in sex education. No child needs to be taught about "hormone blockers" (aka puberty blockers). No one is "assigned" a sex at birth. We are each either male or female from the moment of conception.

Under the guise of sex ed, children are being taught to memorize, recite, and believe the gender ideology liturgy.

Remarkably little of the so-called National Sex Education Standards document is actually sex ed. It's closer to brainwashing. Most of it force-feeds kids "queer" concepts of gender much like the examples excerpted earlier from the second- and fifth-grade learning targets. And it often begins in the earliest grades.

All this raises a question: why are queer theory adherents so laser-focused on children?

There are multiple reasons why ideological movements target the young. Kids are, by nature, malleable. The very young, in particular, who've had no exposure to alternative ideas, are particularly vulnerable to indoctrination. And when a teacher tells a child, "This is today's lesson—it's what you need to know and you will be tested on it," to a child's mind, it falls under the same rubric as reading, writing, and arithmetic. It's what she or he is in school to learn.

But there's also a darker answer to this question, that can't be ignored. And that goes back to queer theory's roots.

Twentieth-century French philosopher Michel Foucault wasn't queer theory's founder, but his work was a big part of its inspiration.

Among other things, Foucault advocated for abolishing the age of consent—laws that govern the age at which minors can have sex with adults. In Foucault's studies of how European cultures through the ages viewed sexual practices, he noted that the attitudes were inconsistent. Pedophilia was accepted as normal in ancient Greece and Rome, but rejected as deviant by modern European cultures. If what was considered acceptable or taboo varied from one era to the next, that meant to Foucault that there was no such thing as either sexually deviant or normal.

The writer Pat Califia picked up and expanded on some of Foucault's ideas about pedophilia. She claimed that children of any age could make the decision to have sex with adults and might even initiate the sexual encounter. So it was unfair to punish the adults in such situations.

This assertion isn't just repugnant. It's insanely wrong. While prepubescent children are curious about their own bodies and those of others, they are not yet sexual beings. They don't initiate sex. Unless they've been sexually molested, they don't know what a sexual encounter is. Rapists might claim *she was asking for it . . . he was asking for it*, but no child seduces an adult.

Foucault's and Califia's views inspired Gayle Rubin, an American academic, who wrote what became queer theory's founding document and manifesto, *Thinking Sex: Notes for a Radical Theory of the Politics of Sexuality*. (Rubin didn't label what she was writing "queer theory" at the time; another academic, Teresa de Lauretis, provided the moniker for the school of thought a few years later.)

Published in 1984, the same year Foucault died, *Thinking Sex* began by pointing out that Victorian condemnation of kids' masturbating was misguided—a reasonable claim. But after establishing that children didn't need to be quite so shielded from this natural inclination, she got progressively bolder. Many of her complaints were about laws that regulated adults having sex with children. She lamented, for example, any laws that prohibited the private possession of child pornography.

Her protests about society's treatment of sexual transgressors got more fervent as her essay continued, bemoaning the suffering of pedophiles—or as she labeled them, "boylovers"—from society's stigma, merely because of their sexual tastes. And because no one would defend these (in her view) unfairly oppressed souls, "the police have feasted on them."

Nevermind who those "boylovers" were feasting on.

Queer theory's founding document, which forms the basis for much of the sexually related "social justice" rhetoric of today, germinated from a demand to normalize anything considered deviant. That included not only pedophilia but also sadism, masochism, fetishism, bestiality, exhibitionism, voyeurism, incest, and of course, transsexualism (now called transgenderism). Borrowing from Califia's claims that children might initiate sex, Rubin argued that pedophilia could involve "affection, love, free choice, kindness or transcendence." To condemn virtually *anything* sexual, according to Rubin, was equivalent to bigotry on the basis of race or ethnicity.

"A person is not considered immoral, is not sent to prison, and is not expelled from her or his family, for enjoying spicy cuisine," she wrote. True. But if someone prefers little boys to adults, that's quite different from preferring vindaloo to pizza.

The embrace of queer theory as part of the social justice movement transformed sexual deviants, including sexual predators, into "sexual minorities" and members of the oppressed. The social justice warriors of the academic world scrambled to become their champions. No longer were sexual deviants to be seen as scary people you'd call the cops on if they hung around a playground. Now they were virtuous victims.

Queer theory, when promoted to kids and their parents, is prettied up with pastel rainbows and unicorns. What could be more innocent? The charming images and social justice rhetoric obscure the reality of the movement. And that's on purpose.

Rubin's plea for sexual deviants to be seen as "sexual minorities" was brilliant, in a way. All good liberals know they are expected to stand up for minorities. And most now do, usually while having almost no idea what they're actually defending.

But queer theory's less savory aspects occasionally surface in public. A "pedosexual" group in Germany appears to have been instrumental in reducing possession of child pornography in that country from a felony to a misdemeanor. It's now lobbying to lower the age of consent to twelve. In a paper published by Cambridge University Press titled "LGBTQ . . . Z?," an academic posited that "viewing bestiality in the frame of queer theory can give us another way to conceptualize the limitations of human exceptionalism." Zoo-sexuals want to hitch a ride with the social justice movement, too.

Until constituents called in to protest, Congress was all set to write a million dollar check to an LGBTQ center in Pennsylvania that hosts monthly fetish parties. (Ads for the parties tell people to "Come find your next unexpected kink.")

Meanwhile, a Minnesota law to protect people from discrimination based on sexual orientation included this line, to ensure that pedophiles couldn't claim that protected status for themselves: " 'Sexual orientation' does not include a physical or sexual attachment to children by an adult." So why did a "transgender" state representative (a man who identifies as a woman) try to remove that sentence from the law? Deleting it could have allowed pedophiles to argue that they had legally protected sexual orientation status in the state. Due to an uproar, the "trans" state rep backed down. He claimed he never meant to include pedophilia as a protected sexual orientation. But then, why try to remove the language that denied pedophiles such legal protection?

Queer theory, beyond gender ideology, champions the pedophile, the dog-fucker, the sadist, the voyeur, the exhibitionist, all manner of fetishists, and other "sexual minorities" as people who deserve respect and inclusion.

As you read on, bear in mind the Q at the end of LGBT hasn't gotten much if any publicity for its objectives. Those objectives probably aren't shared by your virtue signaling co-worker or your woke relative or your child's social justice warrior fifth-grade teacher. Though they're un-likely to have a clue what queer theory is all about, they are unwittingly abetting its advance. And children are in the cross-fire.

In recent years, in attempts to be inclusive, many school districts have eliminated celebrations for Christmas, Halloween, Valentine's Day, or any holiday that originated from a religion or culture, even if the holi-day decorations—elves, hearts, black cats—are completely separate from whatever first inspired the day of celebration.

So kids might never see a brightly lit evergreen in their auditorium, and they might not get to exchange Valentine cards with classmates. But when it comes to one belief system, the decorations and holiday celebrations seem never to end. This is a partial list of LGBTQ holidays that are promoted in schools and elsewhere, organized by their place on the school calendar:

- October is LGBTQ History Month and includes National Coming Out Day and International Pronoun Day.
- In November, there's Trans Parent Day, Trans Awareness Week, and Transgender Day of Remembrance.
- In February, it's Black Lives Matter at School's Week of Action (three of Black Lives Matter at School's thirteen "Guiding Principles" for schools promote trans ideology and queer theory).
- Transgender Day of Visibility is in March.
- International Day against Transphobia and A-gender Pride Day occur in May.
- June is Pride Month. All month.
- July brings us Non-Binary Awareness Week, International Non-Binary People's Day, and International Drag Day.

Every one of these gets celebrated somewhere. Maybe at your kids' schools? And yes, young kids are being taught that the belief system behind all these holidays is based on fact.

Trans swag adorns countless public and private schools, and not just on one of the specially designated days, weeks, or months. In some schools, trans paraphernalia is ever present, draped on the walls, covering the windows, and pinned on the bulletin boards. Signs remind students to respect others' pronouns before many of them are old enough to have learned what a verb, noun, or adjective is.

Pride Month is the biggie. Schools are awash with images of trans unicorns, "genderbread" men, and pastel rainbow-color flags. Those doing the decorating will tell you that it's all about inclusivity, and maybe they believe it. But isn't it likely that, instead of being inclusive of gender-confused kids, they're creating the confusion?

In Los Angeles, National Coming Out Day has been expanded into a Week of Action for kids as young as pre-K. For Pride Month, Chicago Public Schools created a video on which the educators and principals announced their pronouns while one gave a shout-out "to the non-binary young people in Chicago and all my best sexuals!" In Portland, a school counselor who is also a drag performer helped organize an elementary school festival with a drag show, drag queen story time, and a gender-affirming Q&A. (The Portland event was canceled after the school got inundated with angry calls and emails.)

Psychotherapist Grace Ellison says that while it might be difficult to persuade an adult to identify as trans who didn't choose that route for him or herself, you can absolutely convince a child to claim a transgender identity. "You can create any type of child you want. That's the whole point. They're very moldable and malleable at that age."

Choose your own gender, your own pronouns, and demand that everyone call you by an opposite sex name! If mom and dad won't go along, they're unsafe. Parents are the enemy.

Trans kids are cool kids.

Raef Haggag was born and raised in Montgomery County, Maryland. He's always loved the area, and had always been happy with the school system. His seven-year-old daughter was a first-grade student in the local public school, and until recently, he had every reason to expect he'd be sending his toddler son there, too, once the boy was old enough.

So, he was stunned when school administrators cavalierly decided to teach all public school children in Montgomery County lessons based on LGBTQ ideology (emphasis on the TQ), without parental consent, without adequate notice, and without the right to opt out.

He and a number of other parents bought copies of the books the school system planned to add to the curriculum and compared notes on what they found.

One book, for pre-kindergarteners, was about what kids would see at a Pride parade; it instructed them to search for images among the parade revelers for, among other things, a drag queen and underwear. Another book, for kindergarten through fifth-grade students, told the story of a boy who identified as a transgender girl and whose mother made him a wig so he'd look more feminine. Yet another for the same age group was about the sexual attraction one girl felt for another.

"I think it's important for parents to talk to their kids about these issues because there are people in our community, there are people in our society that identify as trans," says Haggag. "But children should not be exposed to the idea that you should be able to explore your gender identity. That is not based in any science. That is not based in any factual understanding. That is, in many ways, a religious belief, if you will."

Haggag says he has no problem with other people believing what they want. But what they can't do, or shouldn't be able to do, is impose their beliefs on others, especially on impressionable children in a public school system.

"From a strictly freedom lens, the freedom to teach your children the values that you want them to have, this is where I think it's very problematic."

Before deciding to pursue his passion as a singer-songwriter full-time, Haggag taught high school computer science. His wife was still teaching in the school system at the time the Pride books mandate came down, but has since quit (they now plan to homeschool).

Both the Haggags had a good grasp of what rights parents were supposed to have, which included the legal right to opt their children out of sex education lessons. And lessons involving books on gender transition and sexual attraction certainly qualified as sex-related, even if they're not what most parents would view as education.

But Montgomery County was not just ignoring those legal rights. Decision-makers had actively schemed to subvert them. Instead of using the books in sex education classes, which would have been optional, the titles were made an intrinsic part of the English Language Arts curriculum. English Language Arts classes, unlike sex education, were mandatory. The Supreme Court has since ruled: parents can opt out.

Dr. Erica Anderson was born a male, identifies as a transgender woman, but is not an ideologue. The clinical psychologist often provides expert testimony in court cases, explaining why it's wrong for schools to affirm alternate sexualities and genders in children without their parents' knowledge or consent. It should be noted that Anderson does not entirely oppose adolescents adopting new gender identities in all instances. But, he says, kindergarten is much too young to introduce such concepts, pointing to an expansive amount of research that shows children are developmentally incapable of fully grasping what the schools imagine they're teaching them. "I think some of these school districts start jumping the gun and going way too far in their curricula." In his view, forcing the Pride picture books on kids went too far.

At my request, psychotherapist and clinical supervisor David Habib

Martin LPC reviewed the book *What Are Your Words: A Book About Pronouns*, one of the picture books that Montgomery County Public Schools chose for Pride Month story hour (schools are "Reading the Rainbow" with a different LGBTQ book getting read to children every day during the month of June). This one was meant to be read to children in grades K–3. In it, a five-year-old boy spends an entire afternoon trying to decide whether he wants his pronouns to be she/her, they/them, ey/eir or something else. All the adults he meets as he walks through town with his trans-identifying uncle (or is it actually his aunt?) eagerly ask the little boy what his "words" are and also announce their own pronouns.

I wondered about the developmental appropriateness of this particular book for this age group. I also asked about other psychological effects on children of reading such books.

"Above all, pseudo-pronouns have no place in young minds that are still learning rules of language, much less because these are arbitrary and fictitious labels and terms," he replied. He added that indoctrination was quite obviously a "shameless and aggressive" goal of the text. "This is the mechanism by which religions and ideology work on the implicit memory and cognitive foundation of children."

Therapist Stephanie Winn also agreed to read and analyze picture books from Montgomery County's LGBTQ library. The first, *Jacob's Room to Choose*, begins in a kindergarten classroom, when the teacher asks if anyone needs to use the bathroom. The text explains that Jacob and Sophie have raised their hands, and it shows their images: one child wears a green dress and has shoulder-length blonde hair; the other child, whose hair is somewhat shorter, is wearing khakis and a plaid shirt. It isn't until the next page, when he gets to the door to the boys' room, that children reading along will learn that Jacob is the one in the dress.

Inside the boys' bathroom, the text explains, two boys stare at Jacob, so Jacob runs out without using the toilet. The book suggests that this makes Jacob a victim. But is he?

"[His parents] let him wear dresses in public and expected the world to change around him," says Winn. "That's a very narcissistic thing to do because it's not respecting that we have these heuristics for a reason. We can clock someone's sex easily for a reason and bathrooms are segregated by sex for a reason. I actually think if you have a five-year-old boy who likes to wear pink and wear dresses, that you create space at home for that. It's fine to play with costumes. But I don't think it's wise to send him out in public that way. I think you're inviting bullying and you're inviting other people to abuse him because there aren't so many visible sex differences between children at that age."

Another Pride picture book Winn reviewed was called *My Rainbow*, intended to be read to children in grades K–2. The book begins with happy images of a black family—a mom sitting in a chair, three smaller children playing on the floor with toys and dolls, while an older boy plays the cello. The text tells the K–2 class that the kid in the dress playing with stuffed animals and dolls is named Trinity and that Trinity is autistic. Trinity pays particular attention to the long hair of one doll and begins to express distress because Trinity's own hair is short. The children *My Rainbow* is being read to have been hearing the word "she" when Trinity is mentioned. But on page seven, it gets super confusing for the average first-grader, after Trinity complains about not having long hair.

The mom points to her own short hair and tells Trinity that short hair is fine for girls.

But Trinity wasn't persuaded.

"I don't think you understand, Mom. I'm a transgender girl . . . People don't care if cisgender girls like you have short hair. But it's different for transgender girls."

In other words, Trinity is actually a boy. How are children in kindergarten through second grade supposed to understand that? Most won't recognize the terms "transgender" and "cisgender." And the book's text doesn't explain either word.

"One of the messages that's obviously very insidious and very intended is that a transgender girl is a type of girl," says Winn.

They might not yet know what "transgender" means, but children learn that if a purportedly transgender five-year-old wants something, the whole family must stop everything else they're doing and focus on fulfilling that desire. That's the thrust of most of the book: the older sibling and Trinity's parents put their heads together to get Trinity long hair. Family members decide that nothing in the wig store is good enough, so Trinity's mother stays up all night weaving a rainbow-colored wig. Though it's the mom who overcomes obstacles to fulfill a quest, she is treated simply as a supporting character. Trinity, in the new rainbow wig, is the center of attention and is somehow both the book's victim and the hero. This, by the way, is true of all the books: the kid is subtly presented as both victim and hero. And while others go out of their way to get these victims what they imagine they need, it's the presumed victim who, despite not accomplishing anything, is celebrated in the end.

The book's illustrator rendered the wig in pastel rainbow colors that are nearly identical to the transgender version of the pride flag. That almost certainly wasn't coincidence, says Winn. Rainbows, unicorns, mermaids—these are recurring themes in the trans materials marketed to children. Children, of course, find such images charming and disarming, as they're meant to.

I asked her about the mandate to "Read the Rainbow" every day to little kids for the entire month of June—Pride Month. What effect might that have on children in the schools that did this? Her response suggests that parents like the Haggags were right to be concerned.

"Overall, it sends a message that this is really, really important," says Winn. "It's really a strong ad campaign. It's just shy of telling kids overtly, 'This is what we want for your future.'"

A number of teachers and principals in the Montgomery County school district also wrote to the school board that the books were troubling, noting hidden agendas and attempts at indoctrination.

The problems they cited went beyond the books themselves. They objected to directives that would force them to teach the ideology as fact. Those directives came in the form of talking points meant to override any objections children might have about the books' confusing messages.

For example, if a child were to say about the transgender concepts in the books, "That's weird. He can't be a boy if he was born a girl," the teacher was instructed to scold the child for making "hurtful" comments.

If a child, confused by language and images in the books that made it difficult to discern a character's sex should ask, "Is that a boy or a girl?" the teacher was told to counter with: "We can't know someone's gender by looking at them. Also, not everyone is a boy or girl."

And if a child were to follow up with the question, "What body parts do they have?" the teacher was directed to respond: **"When we're born, people make a guess about our gender and label us boy or girl based on our body parts. Sometimes they're right and sometimes they're wrong. Our body parts do not decide our gender."** [emphasis added]

Is it any wonder that educators objected? But like the parents' protests, their opposition was largely ignored, or dismissed as evidence of bigotry.

By the way, this claim that people only "guess" gender when a child is born is a common theme. It has been repeated countless times in countless schoolrooms across the country. One picture book that's often used in schools to promote the ideology, *It Feels Good to Be Yourself: A Book about Gender Identity*, includes very similar language that makes an identical point:

> *When you were born, you couldn't tell people who you were or how you felt. They looked at you and made a guess. Maybe they got it right, maybe they got it wrong. What a baby's body looks like when they're born can be a clue to what a baby's gender will be, but not always.*

The now-defunct Project Veritas is a name that no liberal would trust. I admit, when I saw Project Veritas mentioned in a social media post, I was ready to scroll past it. Then I noticed the subject matter. Project Veritas was looking into stealth indoctrination in early elementary to middle school grades, bypassing parents' opt-outs. This was exactly the issue in Montgomery County, Maryland. I had almost decided not to even look because, like most liberals, I was conditioned to view Project Veritas as an operation run by rightwing cranks who could not be trusted.

Project Veritas trained its operatives to use false identities to get close to those it wanted to investigate. It then recorded conversations and meetings when the target of a Project Veritas investigation had his or her guard down. Though it called this journalism, these are more the methods of undercover cops or spies.

What Project Veritas's targets revealed when they believed they were among allies was often devastating when made public. At times, the revelations were merely salacious. At other times, as critics have pointed out, they were misleading. Still, often enough, what Project Veritas investigations turned up included valuable non-public information that people who were affected by the actions of those targets had a right to know.

That was the case when Project Veritas targeted HiTOPS, a nonprofit sex education contractor working in Princeton, New Jersey, schools.

Over a meal shared with undercover Project Veritas operatives, Hi-TOPS employees revealed that they surreptitiously taught gender ideology to children, even when parents had opted their kids out of the classes. Princeton elementary schools hired the contractor to teach a mandatory three-day class in critical race theory, "Pathways to Racial Literacy," but the HiTOPS employees admitted that they sneaked in gender lessons during that time. One of the HiTOPS educators also said the nonprofit's eventual goal was to eliminate opt-outs entirely, but for now, apparently, this was an effective work-around. In another Project Veritas undercover video, a HiTOPS executive revealed what she called "one of the most rewarding experiences."

> We were in the local school system in the elementary school and we were in grades three, four, and five. And, after we were there, five students went to the principal's office and came out.

While the video ends abruptly before we learn what those children "came out" as, these new identities most likely would have been trans, non-binary, or both. Those are the identities that come with new names and pronouns that a school's administrators would need to note on the kids' records.

No one knows how much in-school indoctrination happens by stealth. Parents might learn of it by accident, if at all.

In Colorado, Erin Lee's twelve-year-old, new to her school, was thrilled when her art teacher invited her to join an after-school art club. The invitation was actually a ploy to get the child to join a secret Gender and Sexuality Alliance (GSA) club.

Once at the "art" club, this trusted teacher introduced an outside presenter who volunteered at a "queer" nonprofit. The presenter told the sixth-graders: if you're not 100 percent comfortable with your body, you're trans. (And what child going through puberty is 100 percent comfortable with his or her body?)

This presenter also (incorrectly) told the group that, since the children were now twelve years old, Colorado law would permit them to get prescriptions for puberty blockers and hormones without their parents' knowledge or consent.

The children got one last directive at their bogus art club: don't tell your parents. They might not be "safe." What's said in this room stays in this room.

Other children had been hearing this refrain for a while, and obeying, but Erin Lee's little girl didn't go along. She immediately told her mother what had happened.

Her parents have since sued. Several other parents who had long been kept in the dark about the "art club" and learned of it when Erin Lee went public were shocked to discover what really went on there.

But this queering of the norms is the new normal in so many schools—even in areas not known to be uber-progressive. You might not believe it's happening in your kids' school. You might assume your children would have mentioned something if that were the case. But teachers, counselors, and principals are authorities that kids have been taught they must obey. Are you sure that your child would defy a teacher's direct order to keep such matters secret from you? A famous line from a cult classic film comes to mind. It requires just a slight alteration: *Welcome to the GSA Club. Our first rule is: you do not talk about GSA Club.*

At a California teachers' conference in Palm Springs, "2021 LGBTQ+ Issues Conference, Beyond the Binary: Identity & Imagining Possibilities," two teachers who were speakers bragged about the deceptive tactics they used to recruit kids for a gender-sexuality alliance club. The teacher-presenters obviously assumed that everyone at the conference would be supportive of using any means possible to induct and retain new GSA members. But one attendee leaked a recording of the session to Abigail Shrier. Shrier is the author of *Irreversible Damage*, about the exponential increase in trans identification among teen girls who'd never previously expressed gender confusion.

On the leaked recording, one of the two teachers acknowledged, "We totally stalked what [the students] were doing on Google, when they weren't doing school work" and "Whenever they follow the Google Doodle links or whatever, right, we make note of those kids and the things that they bring up with each other in chats or email or whatever."

One thing they never did was share any information with parents. In fact, they told the conference attendees that they purposely kept no records of who attended their GSA club meetings, so that if a parent asked, they could feign ignorance.

The leaked conference recordings were eye-opening for Jessica Konen, a mother in the school district where the two teachers ran their GSA club. Konen had been shocked when her eleven-year-old daughter suddenly declared, seemingly out of nowhere, that she now considered herself a boy. Konen wanted to support her daughter no matter what, and accepted her proclamation at face value. When she learned about the recordings, she realized that it was this "club" that had indoctrinated her child.

She sued. The school settled with Konen for a reported $100,000. And her daughter, in high school as of this writing, has since abandoned the notion that she was born in the wrong body and is back to living as a girl.

Numerous court cases involving schools socially transitioning children without their parents' knowledge are working their way through state and federal courts. Dr. Anderson notes that the claim that hiding a child's social transition from parents protects the children doesn't make sense. "What that's doing is creating a double life for children," Anderson says. "It's teaching children that it's okay to deceive parents."

Social transitioning is also, as you might recall from the first chapter, a way to cement a cross-sex identity in someone who would almost certainly grow out of it. It's "a powerful psychotherapeutic intervention that will substantially reduce the number of children 'desisting' from transgender identity," wrote psychologist Stephen Levine, PhD, in an affidavit for a Wisconsin lawsuit against a school that encouraged children to hide newly adopted "identities" from parents.

Social transitioning, in other words, is a treatment. Teachers and others who are performing these treatments aren't licensed to provide any psychotherapeutic interventions at all, and certainly not the type that can emotionally damage the children treated.

Despite all the false claims that psychotherapy is conversion therapy when used to explore gender disorders, it's actually social transition that qualifies as true conversion therapy.

It can have numerous effects on children, but protection isn't among them.

Dr. Anderson points out that parents and teachers used to act as partners in children's education. It's bizarre that the official policy in some schools requires them to sever the parent-teacher relationship, and put the parent-child relationship in jeopardy.

Most parents assume that what their kids are being taught today is much the same as what they were taught in school. That assumption leaves children open to indoctrination—and worse—on a massive scale.

Chapter 5

Watch Out Kids,
Your Parents Aren't "Safe"

*"It ain't what you don't know that gets you into trouble.
It's what you know for sure that just ain't so."*

—Mark Twain

Kim Zucker* is a social worker in a large suburban school system in the Pacific Northwest. The "woke" policies she has had to work under have put her in a bind. She was horrified when several other school employees seemed positively gleeful that they could secretly distribute free "packers" to gender-confused girls (to imitate a male genital bulge) and "tucking materials" to gender-confused boys (to hide the contours of their genitalia).

"I'm just like, what? These are people's kids," says Kim. As a mother herself, she recognized that this overstepped all kinds of boundaries. But overstepping boundaries has become the norm in her school district.

She would like to find a different job. But it's the Pacific Northwest. Everyone either is a believer in critical social justice ideology, or is too cowed by the social justice warrior majority mindset to speak out.

Most of the younger teachers, counselors, and others in the school system where she works were indoctrinated into social justice ideology at college. "It's like, whatever's the latest, greatest, most edgy thing that they can be for that's progressive, they're on board for it." The older employees? Kim says the schools are trying to push them out, but meanwhile, they hold regular diversity, equity, and inclusion trainings to ensure that everyone knows what they're supposed to believe.

One of the beliefs treated as fact in these DEI trainings is that all the children in the school system have experienced trauma. Every child is presumed to be a victim. Another is that every non-white child, and any child who identifies as a different gender, has been particularly victimized.

"And it is now the teacher's sort of responsibility to care for and love these children because they've been so traumatized or they come from bad homes," says Kim. "It's in their DEI trainings. So once you've kind of indoctrinated the staff, then they're able to weave that into the way they set up their classrooms and the way they relate to students and the way they teach."

One phrase in particular that Kim says is repeated like sacred scripture: protect trans kids. But often, those who school personnel believe they have to protect these gender-confused kids from are their own parents, the people who know them best, who cherish them, and who need to be informed about what's happening to them at school. Parents have the right to help their children work through any mental health issues in a way that coincides with their values. But that doesn't fit the values inculcated into those who work with children in progressive school systems.

"Whatever people's truth is, you have to compassionately affirm them," Kim says. "And if you don't, then you're a horrible person. It's like creating division, you know? And so I don't see it as this really calculated force, at least by most teachers. I think that they really do believe that they are doing the right thing, that they're being kind."

School staff are trained to believe that if they "out" gender-confused children to their parents, those parents will reject their "queer" children. Parents are presumed "transphobic" until proven otherwise. And being "transphobic," in the view of many of these indoctrinated adults, equals being abusive. Parents aren't safe.

The reality is almost always precisely the opposite. In plaintive posts from the website Parents With Inconvenient Truths About Trans, you'll read countless tales about children who were induced, first to identify out of their sex, and then, to renounce their loving families. Their families haven't rejected them; most would move mountains to get them to come back.

Gender-confused kids too often run away at the urging of activists and predators, ending up in shelters, on the street, or with the "glitter families" who seduced them away from the safety of their homes.

Parents will abandon you, these kids are told. *It's better if you abandon them first.*

Naïve adolescents often have no idea what their parents' actual reactions would be to their decisions to identify out of their sex because activists warn them not to share their new "identities" with mom or dad.

Say nothing. Just run away.

With a caring husband, two beautiful children—George* and Rikki*—a comfortable home, two dogs, and two fish, California attorney Erin Friday's life was about as close to the American dream as it could get. An involved parent, Friday helped out with every school trip. She ran school fundraisers. She took photos for the end-of-year celebrations. She knew all her children's teachers, and trusted them implicitly.

The lean attractive brunette had been a Democrat all her life and thought of herself as a typical California liberal.

The year was 2019. Her daughter arrived home with a bunch of other seventh-grade girls. Though on the cusp of their teens now, it seemed like just a moment ago that the most pressing issue in their lives was deciding on the perfect outfits for their American Girl dolls.

But foremost on their minds today was the sex ed class they'd just attended at school.

As the twelve- and thirteen-year-olds chattered animatedly, Friday got her first inkling that maybe she didn't know as much as she'd thought she had known about the school her children attended.

"They sat in my front yard and they all talked about their new labels. They were all lesbian, pansexual, polyamorous," recalls Friday. "And I said,

'Where are you getting this language? What are you talking about?'"

She gently teased them because, at first, it seemed so silly. What did a twelve-year-old know about being "pansexual" or "polyamorous" or really, about any of the categories they were claiming as their new sexual identities.

Instead of laughing along with her, the kids made fun of her. They called her "cis." They dismissed her with "Okay, boomer" and "Karen."

It was more than disrespectful. It was unsettling. Rikki had never been so rude to her mom before. What was the school teaching these kids?

Friday was about to find out. The school invited parents to a presentation about their new sex education curriculum.

An outside sex ed contractor hired by the school gave the talk and slide presentation.

The sex ed contractor displayed a slide with an illustration of a Barbie doll decked out in pink frills on one side, and G.I .Joe on the other. In between these images were less detailed figures that were meant to represent a host of in-between gender variations.

The facilitator listed all the characteristics that were typically male or female, and noted that some people didn't precisely fit these stereotypes. If you didn't exactly conform to the G.I. Joe or Barbie standard, the presenter stated matter-of-factly, you might be one of these in-between genders. Or, you might be one of countless others. *Each person has a unique gender identity!*

Friday couldn't believe how regressive all this was. Whatever happened to the idea that all children could grow up to be whatever they chose to be, unhampered by the creaky old conventions of centuries past?

She had been a tomboy as a child herself. What did that make her?

She raised her hand, a touch of exasperation perhaps evident in her voice: *But there are no G.I. Joes or Barbies*, she said. *Some men like to cook. Some women like to punch a punching bag. If that made them trans, then everyone was trans, right?*

All around her sat other parents who she would have expected to agree with her, and to recognize the absurdity of this talk. Wasn't anyone else alarmed? She knew a number of them. They were school volunteers, Cub Scout leaders, Girl Scout leaders, people who cared about and were involved with their kids. "And they were all sitting there looking at me with icy eyes."

Despite the disapproving response from others in the room, she kept asking questions and pushing back against this unscientific hogwash.

No, absolutely not, she protested when the facilitator said they should introduce themselves to kids by announcing their pronouns and their sexual and gender identities. All any kid needed to know about her was that her name was Erin and she was Rikki's mom. *Why are we teaching kids to adopt these labels?* she asked.

As disturbing as she found the "sex ed" presentation, there was not much she could do about it now. Rikki had been exposed to it before she had. What was done was done.

Friday didn't yet realize how that one class could have so many repercussions.

"I started to notice that there were more girls coming over to my house with long brown hair going by 'they.' And my daughter is saying, *'Oh, you have to call her Sam.'*"

Friday flatly refused. Though it was disconcerting, it was still someone else's kid, not hers. Even when Rikki started wearing big floppy sweatshirts, Friday didn't make the connection. She remembered being a thirteen-year-old girl herself. She'd worn a shirt when she went swimming so no one would see her blossoming female body. It seemed that Rikki was going through something similar.

And then, halfway through eighth grade's second semester, the Covid-19 pandemic hit. Everyone masked. Everything shut down. School moved into the home. There were no extracurricular activities, no class trips. No actual classes. Just Zoom.

Rikki had always been a girlie girl. Artsy, a little quirky, she expressed her creative side through sewing and knitting. Friday was relieved she had an outlet during those long months of lockdown. Boys were getting outside and playing sports but girls sat alone in front of their screens.

"She started to sew costumes that were male characters. And then she would wear a binder so that she'd look like the male character. And again, I kind of thought of it as theater, like, you know, she's doing something. She doesn't do sports. She's doing something that's making her happy."

Rikki redecorated her room in dark emo and goth style. That long beautiful brown hair that had danced so prettily in the breeze got chopped into a short spiky do. It looked awful to Friday but she recalled her own teen years, how she'd gotten a ghastly perm in an attempt to look like a rocker. "A lot of us did crazy things when we were in high school trying to individualize, trying to figure out who we were." Rikki didn't seem to be doing anything so different.

But her daughter had also become sullen and snippy. The teen didn't want to eat dinner with the family any more. Friday chalked it up to the combined stresses of Covid isolation and puberty. The friends Rikki did see in person were off-putting, to say the least. One girl was tattooing herself and her mom was fine with it. Friday felt total angst about these companions but choices were limited. She let it go.

The new school year began as the old one had ended: in Covid lockdown. Rikki was now a freshman in high school, but everything was still virtual. She was attending a school she had never yet physically entered.

Friday's home office was right down the hall from her daughter's room. "I heard her on her school computer being referred to by the teacher with a male name."

What the heck? When she asked Rikki to explain, the teen said: *"I'm a boy."*

At first, the bewildered mom didn't register what her child meant. *"What are you talking about? No, you're actually a girl."*

And then, all the little things Rikki had been doing that hadn't quite made sense took on a disturbing meaning: Rikki believed she was trans.

Those male TV character costumes Rikki had been designing, sewing, and wearing? She wasn't simply cosplaying. She was creating an alternate version of herself, a new person.

But why on Earth was the school playing along? Friday called and demanded to know.

"I actually thought the teachers would be on my side," she says. "I thought the school would be on my side. I thought the doctors would be on my side. I thought if I could just explain: *'Look, she's depressed. Covid was really hard on her. She was a girlie girl. Like, her room was filled with My Little Pony. Like, none of this is true.'* I didn't know that they were going to look at me as a horrible human until I made that phone call."

The school administrator she spoke with insisted that the school needed to be a "safe place," as if to say that home, where she lived with her parents, was too dangerous a place for these secrets to be revealed.

Nobody working at the high school had even met the new freshman. They knew almost nothing about her, her family, or her home. But if Rikki said she was a boy, as far as the school was concerned, that's what she was. Anyone who said otherwise was "unsafe."

It wasn't long after that call that Child Protective Services (CPS) showed up at Friday's door, along with the police. The CPS social worker said they came knocking because Rikki had Googled: *How many Monster drinks would it take to kill a 110-pound person?*

How could CPS have information about what her daughter was searching for on the web? Because the school had it. The school provided all the kids with iPads. And the school monitored their searches.

"You don't get to know, mom and dad, but the school gets to know what your kid is looking at on the Internet. Isn't that interesting? What country are we living in? The school is spying on your child."

At least CPS didn't open a file on the family. When government agencies routinely back altering the gender of even the smallest children, that can be a real danger. Loving parents around the country have lost custody for the crime of not believing that their children had magically swapped sex. Friday thinks it might have helped that she mentioned, several times, that she was a lawyer.

It was time to go into warrior mom mode. She removed George and Rikki from the public school system that had introduced the ideology. She enrolled them in Catholic school, instead. It wasn't a perfect fix. Even in Catholic school, her son was exposed to critical race theory-laced lessons, but it was better.

She began to put the puzzle pieces together, in an effort to understand how such a feminine child could imagine herself a boy. Critical race theory had to be a big part of it, she realized. "When your parents are married and you have a car in the driveway and you go on vacation and you've never missed a meal and you have your own bathroom—these are all points for being an oppressor. How do you get out of that?"

She could see how claiming to be trans might appeal to her sensitive, compassionate child. It allowed her to escape the guilt. She would instantly become a member of the oppressed, a victim rather than a victimizer.

Searching Rikki's phone, Friday, at first, found nothing suspicious. It took a while to discover that her daughter had a whole other set of accounts under an alias.

Those accounts opened the door to a dark world that Friday barely knew existed. Some messages were from Rikki's real-life friends but most were from strangers she'd met on social media. They told her that her parents were bigots and homophobes.

Emancipate. Run away, these new online "friends" insisted. They warned that if her parents discovered her online exchanges, they could take her phone; if they did, that was child abuse.

An ugly theme ran through many of these messages, echoing what the school administrator had implied: if her parents wouldn't accept her adopted gender, they weren't safe to be around.

"So, tell a girl going through puberty, everything from the way you move, talk, your arms, your genitals, your waist, your feet, your hands: they're all wrong. You, child, were born wrong. And your parents hate you. That's transgenderism."

That wasn't the worst of it.

Friday scrolled through this new-to-her world of social media—Instagram, Twitter, Discord, even Pinterest. Strange men had been reaching out, attempting to seduce her daughter. It was terrifying.

"Once these kids say that they're trans online, it's like a beacon, a calling card for pedophiles," says Friday. "I got into her phone and I saw the messages and the amount of porn that was sent to her from older people. The telephone numbers, I called them. I looked up their accounts. They were grown men."

Older girls on social media coaxed the younger ones to sell semi-nude pictures of themselves to these pedophiles.

"You're not going to have breasts anyway when you transition. So, you might as well just show them and get money for them."

Friday was relieved that Rikki didn't go along. Her daughter had actually been the voice of reason, telling other young girls, don't do it.

"I know these kids did it because I went to the police," she explains. "And the police said I didn't have a cause of action because my child didn't do it."

Erin Friday's entire life became centered around keeping Rikki safe. That meant watching everything she did. It was a risk, because Rikki was already depressed, already feeling isolated due to Covid lockdowns, and now, her mom was invading her privacy and banishing every friend who was involved in the trans craze.

Friday confiscated her phone. She took away her access to the internet entirely, except for during Zoom classes, which she sat in on. It was awful for both of them but she was on a mission. Her daughter was going to grow up healthy—with all body parts intact. That was what mattered.

"I had to take the hate that she was giving me," she says. "I had to take the risk that she may never talk to me again. She may hate me forever. But I had to fight."

She says there were days when she wanted to quit and say, *Go do it. Be trans. Go do it.* But she stuck it out.

"The most disgusting part of all of it is that the world is cheering your child on. So basically, you're watching your child die by a thousand cuts and everybody's cheering her on and looking at you as the demonic one."

Though she kept a near-constant vigil, she couldn't keep watch every second. She'd toss Rikki's room and find chest binders and old iPhones that her banned friends somehow passed along to her. She'd throw them out. More would appear.

"It's almost like they're a drug addict and you need to get the heroin out of their room. You need to make sure that they have no money, and track where they are."

Because Rikki would become angry when anyone called her by her birth name, Friday started using nicknames, or terms of endearment—anything but the made-up male name.

"Then I would throw in her real name and let it sit and see if it exploded her, which it didn't." She started dropping Rikki's "dead name" into conversation two or three times a day, without making a big deal of it, almost as if it were an accident.

"I had this long conversation with her about social contagions. And she would name one and then I would name one. And then at the end, I said, 'Well, people think gender identity is a social contagion.' And I walked away."

She didn't push it. The goal was to get her daughter to think. And Rikki did seem to be thinking. Friday believed, or at least hoped, that the girl was beginning to see the cracks in the ideology.

Fall gave way to winter and the holiday season. The family had a beach trip planned for Christmas. Rikki had previously bought boy's swim trunks and Friday said nothing. Instead, when it came time to pack, she laid out all the bathing suits so the kid could choose what she wanted to bring. It was quite a selection: a tankini, a one-piece, the boy shorts, and Friday's own white bikini that Rikki used to like to play dress-up in when she was younger.

And that's the one Rikki put on—the white bikini.

Friday tried to be cool but her heart was bursting. She made an off-hand comment that it looked so good on Rikki, she would never again be able to wear it herself. She couldn't make a big deal about Rikki wearing something so classically female, or the teen might revert.

As Rikki walked downstairs, Friday texted her husband. "*She's wearing the white bikini. Don't say anything.*"

"And that was when we knew she was coming back."

It didn't happen all at once. After vacation, Rikki began wearing big sweatshirts again. And then, she'd show up in girl clothes. Back and forth. Her parents continued to play it cool, but stopped using nicknames and called Rikki by her own name again, more confident now that their daughter was beginning to accept herself. She again became the loving girl she'd always been before the trans phase. Her depression started to lift, and the belief that she'd been born in the wrong body resolved along with it.

Has Rikki completely abandoned the ideology?

"I can't answer that," says Friday. "She herself does not believe that she's trans. She does not believe that she's a boy. She knows that she's a female. Does she believe still that there are trans people out there? Like there's that 'true trans' or there are people born in the wrong body? I don't know. She's still a minor. She doesn't want to have the conversations with me about it. It's a dark time in her life. It's a dark time in our family's life."

But Rikki did thank her mother. And she tells her mother she loves her, every day.

Erin Friday is today a fierce fighter against the belief system that nearly took her child away from her. As the co-lead of the US chapter of Our Duty, she campaigns for new legislation to protect children from the predatory ideology taught in schools across her state and around the country.

"Once I got out of my sorrow and my daughter was stable mentally, I decided that I needed to be an advocate. No one was coming in to save us. I really thought that the world would figure this out. I thought that there would be rational minds. I waited and waited. And then I said, no one's coming. No one's helping us. We've got to do this on our own."

When she was an eighth-grader, Sage Blair of Appomattox, Virginia, an artistic but deeply troubled teen, told her grandmother, Michele—who had adopted her when she was tiny and thus was legally her parent—that all the girls in her class claimed to be bi, trans, or lesbian. Michele isn't sure when, but Sage eventually followed the crowd, opting for a new "identity," possibly while she was hospitalized in a psychiatric hospital that summer.

When she started high school, Sage's school counselor was eager for Sage to embrace a cross-sex identity. But the counselor told Sage that the other girls weren't comfortable sharing the girls' bathroom with someone who identified as a boy, so she should use the boys' bathroom, instead. Sage told the counselor that the boys bullied her when she did so, and several threatened to rape and otherwise harm her. But the school kept most of this information, including Sage's male name (Draco), from her grandparents.

Eventually, it all came out, and her grandparents promised she wouldn't have to go back to the school where she was being tormented. But that same night, Sage escaped through a window and ran away, leaving a note for her grandparents that said she loved them.

The teen—petite, frail, and under 100 pounds—was immediately abducted by a stranger. He drugged and violently raped the fourteen-year-old virgin in the backseat of his car. He then took her to Washington, DC, where he passed her around to several other men.

A week later, the FBI tracked the missing girl to a locked room in the Baltimore home of a registered sex offender. Once law enforcement rescued her, they contacted Michele and her husband Roger to let them know where they could come to pick her up the following morning.

The nightmare should have ended there.

Anyone with half a heart and a functioning brain would do everything possible to quickly reunite a brutalized child with the family members who loved her, right?

But between the time Sage was rescued and the following morning, when Michele and Roger were scheduled to pick her up, the court appointed a public defender to represent Sage. And once that legal representative heard the magic word "transgender," all bets were off. Michele and Roger had referred to Sage as Sage. That made them non-affirming and "abusive" in the public defender's eyes; she got child protective services to open an investigation into the Blairs.

While the Blairs fought to regain custody of their child, the Maryland court placed the diminutive girl in a juvenile detention center. A boys' juvenile detention center, of course, to match Sage's assumed male identity.

The boys she was housed with sexually assaulted her. Much later Sage would tell her grandparents (who had been desperately fighting to get her home) that no one had told her they were battling the legal system to regain custody. She said, instead, that one of the people in Maryland actually claimed that her parents didn't want her any more and that she was going to be placed with a Maryland family who would "affirm" her male identity.

So, again, Sage ran away. And predictably, a predator awaited. He lured her to Texas. There, he raped her. He starved her. He tortured her.

This time it was months before law enforcement found and rescued her. As soon as they did, they contacted Michele who flew out to Texas to get her.

Sage, at last, was back in Virginia, but the harrowing experience left her in need of round-the-clock psychiatric treatment.

And yet, it could have been worse.

What if, instead of being lured to Texas, it had been a "blue" state that again refused to return the girl?

Who knows how Sage's story would have ended?

The visible signs of an ideological takeover are everywhere in the Olympia, Washington, school district.

"These children are completely inundated and enveloped with BLM and Pride from the walls, telling what the different identities are, describing what pansexual is, all the different genders," says Alesha Perkins as she holds up a sign that she says she found on a classroom door. It shows a black man with a moustache, wearing a flowered knotted head scarf and a flowered blouse. Behind him is a raised fist. Above is the headline "Trans Affirming," which is number seven of the Black Lives Matter at School's thirteen "Guiding Principles" for schools. The text reads: "Everybody has the right to choose their own gender by listening to their own heart and mind. Everyone gets to choose if they are a girl or a boy or both or neither or something else and no one gets to choose for them."

Perkins says the poster is typical of the propaganda that greets children every day in every school in the district.

Alesha Perkins, whose three children attended school in the district, has become the unofficial spokesperson for parents and teaching staff in the district who are distressed by the agenda pushed by a school board in which three of the five members claim to have trans or queer children.

Parents worry their kids will be ostracized if they go public with their complaints. Teachers worry about their jobs. So they tell Perkins what they've observed and she tells the world. It was Perkins who publicized it when the head of the school board claimed the reason Olympia was cutting fourth-grade band was because it was somehow white supremacist.

You might recall, from the previous chapter, what therapist Stephanie Winn said about what children are likely to take away from the experience of having trans-promoting books read to them each day during Pride month: "It's just shy of telling kids overtly, 'This is what we want for your future.'"

In Olympia, it isn't "just shy" of anything. It's so in-your-face, it's a wonder that any kid comes out of the school system still claiming to be the same sex as when he or she went in.

Through Perkins, I met parents and staff from the Olympia school district who each shared elements of one particularly disturbing story. To protect their privacy, I've changed their names and other identifying details.

By all accounts, ten-year-old Maia Chatterjee* was quintessentially feminine. Charming and sociable, Maia had lustrous, long dark wavy hair that she'd wear in braids or pony tails, set off with ribbons. She enjoyed vivid colors—wearing them and creating art with them. Her parents doted on her, especially Veda*, her mom, who didn't seem to mind that Maia could be a bit bossy at times.

It was 2022 and the free-spirited ten-year-old had developed her first crush. His name was Gerald* and she made no secret of her infatuation. But Gerald's family was moving to Florida soon, and Maia was already feeling the first pangs of loss.

Deirdre Collyer's* daughter Amy* was in the same fifth-grade class as Maia, and the two girls would occasionally play together, so Deirdre and Veda got to know each other.

The girls' teacher, Mrs. Barbara Farmer*, was one of the most popular in the elementary school, but Deirdre had an uneasy feeling about the woman. It began when another friend who had a daughter in the class confided that Farmer seemed to be overstepping boundaries.

"She was really uncomfortable with the way her daughter had started to only want to talk to Mrs. Farmer, like at nighttime or weekends. And so she felt kind of replaced," she recalls.

Deirdre didn't know at the time that her friend's little girl wasn't the only one that Farmer held long after-hours chats with.

Maia's parents hailed from India. Though the family maintained close bonds with the local Indian community and its customs, children aren't always as enthusiastic about tradition as their parents. One day, Mrs. Farmer asked the class what they'd done over the weekend, and Maia said she'd been at a community event, learning to do a traditional Indian dance, and the dress she had to wear was itchy. She didn't like it.

Classmates who overheard the exchange recalled that Mrs. Farmer turned Maia's "itchy" complaint into something else. If Maia didn't like dresses, she said, she shouldn't be forced to wear dresses. Maybe, she continued, Maia's real issue wasn't just one itchy dress but that Maia was being pushed into conforming with a female stereotype that didn't match how she felt inside.

Many months later, from what Veda told Deirdre, Maia revealed to her mother that it was around this time that Mrs. Farmer had begun suggesting to the little girl that she might not be a girl at all.

Mrs. Farmer had her favorites, according to Amy, and Maia was at the top of that list. The ten-year-old and her teacher were often together, chatting away. Those chats didn't end with the school day. They also exchanged after-hours emails.

There was an empty classroom next to Farmer's that the teacher called the "dark room." She designated it as a safe space where kids in her class could go at any time for any reason. No permission needed and no explanation required. They could leave in the middle of a lesson, if they chose to. The only rule Mrs. Farmer made for the dark room was that they had to be quiet.

So children would go there to do homework or read or listen to headphones or just sit by themselves if they needed space.

One day, according to Amy, Mrs. Farmer said, *"I have something to share with you guys. Listen to this."*

And then she read a poem to the class about how a girl can be a boy or a boy can be a girl. Amy and several classmates, uncomfortable with the message, left for the dark room. Sitting in the empty classroom quietly reading their books would have been completely acceptable at any other time. But, for some reason, on this occasion, Mrs. Farmer changed the rules.

"[She] went in there and she told them that they were being inappropriate," says Deirdre. "They were required to participate in this poem."

Cate Bennett's* little boy, Henry, was in the same fifth-grade class as Amy and Maia. His mom had been to Pride events herself, but she balked at Henry sitting through a planned drag queen story hour. She felt that drag queens' burlesque-style vamping was way too sexualized for a ten-year-old. Henry told his mom that, as she'd instructed him to do, he tried to go to the dark room during the story hour. But Mrs. Farmer wouldn't let him. She demanded he stay and listen. Cate was furious.

Something similar happened when the principal, decked out in an inflatable rainbow unicorn outfit, pranced and sang a Pride song at a school assembly. The kids knew what was coming any time rainbows and unicorns were involved, so some of them tried to escape to the girls' bathroom.

Mrs. Farmer was right behind them, says Deirdre. "She made them come in and participate."

But it was a somewhat more ambiguous event that Deirdre now believes precipitated the big change in Maia. Farmer brought her class out to the elementary school garden and told each child to choose a nickname and write it on a wood chip, along with their pronouns. This, she said, would be how they'd address each other at school from now on.

Not long after that, at the end of April, Farmer announced to her fifth-grade class that Maia had adopted a permanent new name and pronouns.

From now on, the children had to call Maia "Felix." And they couldn't call her she. "Felix" would now be using he/him and they/them pronouns.

Also—most important—it was a secret. The children weren't allowed to tell anyone outside the school. Maia's parents couldn't know. And that meant the kids in her class had to keep it secret from *their* parents, too, because if their own parents found out, they might tell Maia's.

Poor little Amy. She couldn't figure out how to talk about Maia in front of her parents. She knew she'd get in trouble with Mrs. Farmer if she didn't call Maia "Felix," but she'd *also* get in trouble if her parents found out from her.

One day while her mother was in the room, she referred to her classmate Maia as "he." She quickly realized it was supposed to be "she" when they were outside of school and corrected herself. But in saying "he," Amy had broken Mrs. Farmer's rule about hiding Maia's new identity from all the parents. Her teacher would be mad at her. With tears in her eyes, she spilled the whole story to her mother. Deirdre was aghast. She told her daughter that she no longer had to participate in the subterfuge. But Amy insisted she did. She had to say it right or she'd get in trouble. Focused on her own little girl's distress, Deirdre didn't stop to wonder whether the idea of claiming a boy's identity had originated with Maia herself. At the time, she had no reason to believe otherwise.

Meanwhile, Farmer had called a meeting at the school to instruct all those who worked at the elementary school on how to hide Maia's "transition" from her parents. Bruce Jeffries*, a member of the school staff, had gotten an email about a week earlier that one of the girls was now to be called a boy. He knew the child and was puzzled. She'd always seemed so girlish. Where had this come from?

Parents were able to log in to the school's system to view all their children's records. At the meeting, Barbara Farmer showed the others how they could input information about students in the school's system in an area that parents couldn't access. That's where "Felix's" name and pronoun change would go, and anything else related to the new identity. One of the other teachers said he wasn't comfortable hiding such pertinent information from parents and wasn't sure if it was even legal to do so.

Bruce says that this teacher was reprimanded for daring to raise questions. "If you didn't follow this, you would be fired," he recalls the teacher being told. "You would lose your teaching certificate. You'd be removed."

The staffers were given a handout that suggested that failing to follow these directives might be illegal under Washington state law and could result in arrest. Aside from the one teacher, Bruce says that no one complained openly about keeping parents in the dark. In fact, the next day, staff emails to Farmer were overwhelmingly positive. *"Oh, that was amazing. We support you. What a great job."*

On Friday, June 3rd, the fifth graders took a walk to the middle school, about a mile away, that they'd attend the following year when they entered sixth grade. Farmer had had her class make tie-dye rainbow shirts and instructed them to wear them and other rainbow attire on their walk, turning it into yet another Pride event. Deirdre was acting as a chaperone, while other parents, including Veda, arrived later to join their children for this right of passage. The 150-acre LBA Park, with its woods, trails, and playground areas, was just a few blocks from the middle school. After their tour, the group stopped to play in the park before heading back to the elementary school, settling for a while in a field next to the woods with two baseball diamonds.

One boy shouted out to Maia, "Hey, Felix," and Maia answered, apparently without thinking. Veda was startled. Then another boy used the secret name, and Veda demanded, *"Why are you calling her that?"*

At that moment, "Somebody came and talked to Mrs. Farmer," says Deirdre. "It got kind of hush, hush, quiet, and I tried to walk towards them . . . You could tell something was going on."

Without a word to the parents, Farmer rounded up the kids and they all took off into the surrounding woods. Veda raced after them.

"I mean, here we are, the chaperone parents that are supposed to be hanging out and having this experience together. And we're all sitting in the park just going, 'Where'd they go? Where are they?' We tried texting and calling. They wouldn't answer . . . It was very strange. I've never had a teacher that had parent helpers not communicate with their parent helpers and isolate the kids from them, and then, just be gone for that amount of time. I'm like, *Where's my child, and who are you to take my child?*"

The teachers and students reappeared after about forty minutes, with no explanation of where they'd gone or why.

When they did, Veda wasn't with them.

Weeks went by. It was June 22nd, the last day of the school year. Deirdre wondered why Maia didn't show up for a neighborhood get-to-gether to celebrate. When Amy told her mom that Maia hadn't been in school for weeks, Deirdre became concerned.

So she reached out to Veda via text. "And I just said . . . 'It sounds like you guys have been going through a lot in your family. And I just wanted to let you know, no judgment, no nothing. We're here for you. You're not alone. And if you ever want to talk, you can.' And then she's like, 'Can I call you?'"

The story Veda shared was deeply unsettling.

Veda said she believed that Mrs. Farmer was trying to take Maia away from her and her husband, and the parents worried that the school might have the power to do it. It was run by the government. They were from another country. They felt threatened.

If all this sounds like paranoia, it won't in a moment. Emails from Mrs. Farmer, obtained via a public records request, suggest that the threat was very real.

After the boys called her daughter by her secret male name, Maia told her mom everything. The main reason Maia was calling herself "Felix" was to please the teacher who had showered so much attention on her. But she didn't want to be a boy any longer. Still, she was worried that if she stopped: *"The teacher is going to be so mad at me and she's not going to like me."*

Emails in the public records cache suggest that Veda approached Mrs. Farmer that same day.

The mother and daughter walked into the school holding hands. When Mrs. Farmer saw them, at first, she was warm and inviting. Then Veda confronted her: *"What are you doing with my daughter?"*

"Mrs. Farmer stopped even acknowledging the mom and would

only look at her daughter," says Deirdre. *"Are you okay?"* Mrs. Farmer asked Maia as she leaned in closer to the girl, speaking to her almost as if she were a hostage. *"Do you need help?"*

Stunned by the way the teacher was behaving, Veda demanded, *"Stop talking to my daughter. Leave her alone."*

But Farmer kept on speaking in that same tone, only to the girl, not acknowledging Veda's presence at all. To Veda's ear, Farmer's message to her child was clear: say the word, and Farmer would "help" her escape her family.

Furious, Veda decided to lodge a complaint against Farmer with the principal. She got nowhere. The principal and school counselor backed up the teacher—again, treating the mom like *she* was the problem.

"Veda felt like, as a parent, she had no rights or power," says Deirdre. "And then it scared her because these American schools, like can the government really do this with my child without me knowing?"

The shaken parents immediately took Maia and her younger brother to what they described to friends as a "safe house" in Oregon.

But the teacher wouldn't leave Maia alone. She emailed the child a number of times over the next few weeks beginning, innocently enough, on June 10th, with an email saying, "We miss you" and "Can anyone swing by and talk to you or your mom and help?" A few days later, she sent another short email. Maia didn't respond to either. Farmer sent a third on June 17th and the fifth-grader finally replied, saying that her family was moving. The little girl was quite upset that she wouldn't get to see her friends at school again or even get to say good-bye. And she was scared of going to a new place where she didn't know anyone and might not be accepted.

Although Maia's emails focused on keeping in touch with classmates and worrying that she'd lose her school email address, Farmer's were different in tone and content. Some read like messages from a creepy stalker. Nine out of the eighteen that Farmer sent to the child on June 18th either disparaged Maia's family, tried to undermine her parents, or promoted the trans identity that Maia had already at this point abandoned. Another seven of those eighteen looked suspiciously like love-bombing, constantly telling the child how much she was missed.

When Maia mentioned that she'd been visiting relatives since leaving school, Farmer wrote: "Glad you weren't just home," as if to say that home wasn't a good place to be. Less than a minute later, Farmer sent another email that again appeared to be an attempt to undermine the child's relationship with her parents: "I kept emailing you but I worried your mom interfered before you saw my messages :("

Another followed the same theme: "Is there anyone at all who is safe in your family? Or a neighbor?"

Maia didn't respond to any of these, and never suggested she agreed with Farmer's negative remarks about her family. She also didn't respond to an email the teacher sent with the phone number for the Trevor Project, which Farmer told her to write down somewhere and keep safe. The Trevor Project is one of the main promoters of transgender ideology to teens. It's known for pushing the idea of hiding trans identities from parents.

After encouraging the child to set up a private email account so they could stay connected, the teacher again tried to undermine Maia's relationship with her mother with this message: "Make sure this email is deleted too when we are done bc otherwise when your mom looks, you will be outed instantly."

The ten-year-old didn't acknowledge any of these messages, but Farmer wasn't done. At 5:38 p.m. on June 18, 2022, she made the most blatant attempt to separate the child from her family—and the wording of the email strongly suggests that this wasn't the first time she'd proposed that the child should run away from home: "I was also serious that I would take you into my own home anytime you need. Never think you have no one. You were part of this class for a reason."

The fifth-grade teacher signed all these emails, "Barb."

Farmer was right in assuming that Veda would "interfere," as she put it. The loving and now desperate mother read every one of the messages and showed several to Deirdre and other friends. They appear to be a big part of the reason why Veda and her husband concluded that there was no safe place in this country for their daughter as long as Barb Farmer was able to reach her.

The Chatterjees sent their two children, Maia and her younger brother, to India with the kids' grandparents. The parents stayed in the country long enough to disengage from their jobs and put their house on the market. Though they briefly considered taking action against the school and the teacher, they decided to leave the whole sordid incident behind them—but they gave their friends in the United States permission to share their story.

Meanwhile, apparently unaware that Maia had left the country, Farmer sent one more email on June 24th, inviting the girl to meet her to pick strawberries at a nearby farm. According to what Veda told Deirdre, the mom worried that if Maia were still in the United States and had met the teacher that day, she and her husband might never have seen the girl again.

Was she right?

In 2022, when Barb Farmer was telling Maia that *"I would take you into my own home anytime you need,"* she couldn't have legally hidden the child from her parents. But by May 2023, if she'd persuaded Maia to leave home, she could, indeed, have kept the child's whereabouts secret. Washington Governor Jay Inslee signed a bill into law that would allow a person like Farmer to take Maia and not give her back, so long as that person could cite "compelling reasons." Here's how Washington state law defines "compelling reasons":

" *'Compelling reasons' include, but are not limited to . . .*

(ii) When a minor is seeking or receiving protected health care services.

(d) 'Protected health care services' means gender affirming treatment."

Farmer, meanwhile, even as I write this, is working in the Olympia, Washington, elementary school system as a teacher, and as far as anyone knows, is still fully supported in her actions by the school's leadership.

Chapter 6

Watch Out Parents:
No One, Nowhere, and Nothing Is Safe

"It's terrifying that they're calling it 'gender-affirming care'
when it's really childhood mutilation, before you have the ability
to figure what permanent means."

—Bill Maher

Jamie Reed was a true believer. She referred to herself as a "queer" woman, politically to the left of Bernie Sanders. Her spouse, a woman, identified at the time as a "transman" (she has since detransitioned). On paper, Jamie must have looked like the perfect match for the Washington University Pediatric Transgender Center in St. Louis, Missouri—a clinic set up to dose children with powerful experimental drugs that would either halt puberty's progress or cause the children's bodies to develop features that simulate those of the opposite sex.

When, in 2018, Jamie became the case manager for the clinic, she believed the team would be doing heroic work treating children who had "gender dysphoria." She expected the team would provide whatever the kids needed to lead happy lives as their authentic, cross-sex selves.

At the clinic, Jamie conducted the initial interviews. First talking to the parents, she would find out the child's medical and mental health history, ask when the child "came out" as trans, and what their goals were.

"I felt like it was a very clear-cut protocol that was being followed. I felt like it was based on extensive historical science and research and was the right form of treatment ... I felt like we were not going to be pushing people one way or the other."

Four years after she took the job, this former true believer, deeply distressed by what she'd seen happening to children who came to the pediatric gender clinic, became a whistleblower. She submitted an affidavit to the state's attorney general detailing the clinic's total lack of guardrails. In that affidavit, she shredded the façade of careful treatment.

Along with a psychologist, a psychiatrist, a nurse, and an endocrinologist who prescribed the drugs, the Washington University Pediatric Transgender Center employed an adolescent medicine doctor whose role was supposed to involve working with kids who had questions but didn't want hormones or puberty blockers. After a while, though, that doctor decided that she, too, wanted to prescribe.

With all the doctors on board the child chemical transition train, all the children visiting the center got the same diagnosis and the same treatment, no matter what their underlying issues might be.

Feeling awkward or uneasy because you don't fit in with your peers? You're trans. If you're a tomboy, you're trans. If you're a boy who's better at math than football, you're trans. If other kids bully you, it's because you're trans. If you can't get the attention of the opposite sex, you're trans. If you're same-sex attracted, you must be trans. If you dislike anything at all about your developing body, it means you're trans.

It's unsurprising that kids with mental and emotional health issues— borderline personality disorder, autism, depression, anxiety, ADHD, PTSD, OCD, eating disorders—would be relieved to hear there's an instant cure for whatever ails them. Become a facsimile of the opposite sex. Or just be no sex at all. But medical professionals are supposed to know there is no such thing as a universal cure-all elixir.

From 2020 to the time Jamie Reed left in 2022, the clinic prescribed cross-sex hormones and puberty blockers to more than 600 children. Almost every child who walked through the doors walked out with a prescription for some form of body-altering chemicals. According to Jamie, even children who never asked for puberty blockers or cross-sex hormones got them anyway.

About three-quarters of the patients were girls.

Even if you're persuaded that children should be free to make decisions that permanently alter their bodies, what about children who can't think clearly? Should they be making such choices?

What about the mentally ill boy who was forced by his parent to cross-dress? Jamie says that he got female hormones. What about the girl who just wanted to be sure she wouldn't get pregnant? Instead of birth control, she got male hormones.

"We had a couple patients who believed they were blind," says Jamie. "And yet, they could see. We had a few patients who believed they couldn't walk. But they could. We had a number of patients who then also said that they believed that they had multiple personalities."

These children had lost touch with reality. They needed, at minimum, exploratory talk therapy. Some, perhaps, might have benefited from antipsychotic medicine.

What the clinic prescribed instead were puberty blockers and cross-sex hormones. Yes, for all of them.

Jamie says that most of the kids on hormones had near-constant abdominal pain. One suffered liver damage. Girls on testosterone complained that their clitorises had grown so large, they chafed against their clothes when they walked.

And the treatments often made kids' mental health problems worse. And some of the physical changes caused by the drugs were permanent.

Meanwhile, reluctant parents were coerced into agreeing to these extreme chemical interventions with that terrifying question: *"Would you rather have a dead daughter or a live son?"*

Jamie Reed revealed so many disturbing practices during our interview, it's difficult to say one was more troubling than another. Still, it was particularly chilling to hear that the clinic actively worked to revoke the legal rights of any parent who tried to stand in the way of prescribing such life-altering drugs to their children.

"I remember that I had sent emails to local parent support groups on behalf of the affirming parent," Jamie admits. "And I would say, '*Hey, this mom, you know, gave me permission to share her contact. Can you please reach out with her and help her get set up with an attorney? She needs to sue for legal custody.*'"

Too often, such cases resembled Munchausen-by-proxy. In classic Munchausen cases, a parent or caregiver fabricates tales of disease symptoms in a child so the parent can then bask in the attention from medical professionals. Some might do things to a child that actually makes the child ill. One therapist I interviewed calls this phenomenon "Transhausen." The parent or caregiver either persuades or forces the child to dress and act as the opposite sex. If the other parent tries to safeguard his or her child from forced "transitioning," the "affirming" parent almost always ends up with sole custody.

I asked Jamie the age of the youngest child who was involved in such a custody dispute.

"Five or six," said Jamie. "It was a mom who basically, I think, made her kid be trans."

Jamie says that this little girl's dad fought in court, trying to keep his child from being dosed with experimental drugs. The father did request his little girl's medical records, and if he got all of them, he would have seen Jamie's notes saying that the child didn't actually imagine herself as the opposite sex. "The mom is doing this and the mom's being super creepy and weird."

In any court that saw the child's medical records, Jamie's notation should have been a deal-breaker. But it wasn't. The clinic's doctors testified that the child needed their treatment. About the same time Jamie Reed transferred from the gender clinic to a new job within the same hospital, the little girl was dosed with puberty blockers.

She was eight or nine years old.

Because most family courts limit access to records related to children, there's no way to ascertain how often a "non-affirming" parent loses custody to the parent who wants to transition their child. But a few such cases have gotten media attention.

There was the father in upstate New York who only learned by accident that his ex-wife had been dressing his son in girl's clothing from the time the boy was three years old. He found out when the school sent him a notice with an unfamiliar girl's name. The father fought for the right to keep his child off puberty blockers. He lost.

There was the dad in San Francisco whose ex decided to raise their three-year-old son as non-binary (the mother also identifies as non-binary), and who told the child that he is both a boy and a girl. The dad, who shares custody, says he makes sure the child knows he's a boy.

The story is much the same with a third father whose ex started dressing their son as a girl by age two. He also fought and lost in court. Now, he isn't allowed to even see his child.

You would think that judges would recognize a parent's right to say no to dosing their children with powerful chemicals that can lower IQ, weaken the skeleton, cause organ damage, heart disease, diabetes—all so that children can mimic the opposite sex.

You would think that health-care professionals who claim children were born in the wrong body would have solid evidence to back up their sworn testimony.

You would think . . .

But where gender ideology is involved, you'd be wrong.

As an earlier chapter showed, media play an outsized role in convincing the public at large (which includes the family court judges who rule on such cases) that any child claiming a trans identity actually *was* born in the wrong body, and that the only two choices for that child are "transition" or suicide.

A quick Google search of the terms "gender-affirming" and "life-saving" will yield tens of thousands of results from sources that people rely upon for trustworthy information: CNN, Associated Press, ABC, NBC, CBS, Reuters, *Science Friday*, *Healthline*, the National Institutes of Health, Planned Parenthood, the ACLU . . . and on and on and on.

The consensus is clear. It's a consensus of individuals and organizations that most assume are trustworthy sources. And yet, on transgenderism, they're anything but.

Scientific American might be the most trusted consumer science magazine published today. It's filled with news about the latest scientific discoveries, written in a way that's accessible to the educated non-scientist.

In May 2022, the magazine published an article online titled "What the Science on Gender-Affirming Care for Transgender Kids Really Shows." And then, it republished the same article in March 2023 with an editor's note that it was doing so *"to highlight the ways that ongoing anti-trans legislation is harmful and unscientific."*

It was a repeat of a remarkable piece of trans propaganda.

The article told the story of a forty-year-old married man from Texas using the pseudonym Kelly Fleming. Fleming had recently begun taking cross-sex hormones and had changed his pronouns. Adults have no trouble getting prescriptions for cross-sex hormones in Texas. But he was planning to move to a different state anyway, because Texas has outlawed such drugs for children. We learn that Fleming has two kids, ages twelve and fourteen, both of whom Fleming claims are "agender." The term means that they have no gender at all. Neither actually wants hormones, according to the article, but their father wants to be somewhere they can get them, just in case the kids change their minds.

Back in the 1920s, *Scientific American* made its reputation by debunking medical quackery. That was its claim to fame. A century later, that once august magazine's editors saw nothing questionable in claims about two purportedly gender-free kids whose father imagines himself a woman. No one at the magazine thought to ask the obvious: why on Earth would kids who claim to be sexless need cross-sex hormones?

Cross-sex from what?

The article went on to dismiss any concerns about any of the powerful drugs given to young people. It made the outrageous claim that when kids suffer bone loss after being on puberty blockers, it's just due to lack of exercise (disregarding a Reuters investigation that found that another Texan teen had developed osteoporosis after taking puberty blockers—a disease usually affecting women sixty-five and older that causes the bones to become brittle and break easily). For expert opinion, the article's author relied upon two pediatricians, Dr. Michelle Forcier and Dr. Jason Rafferty, who have since been sued by detransitioner Layton Ulrey for persuading her to take cross-sex hormones despite knowing that she suffered from a plethora of mental health problems that made informed consent impossible.

As icing on the proverbial cake, Forcier is quoted as saying that puberty blockers are "part of the process of 'do no harm.'"

If a parent with a gender-confused child were to go online to seek information from a respected source, this is the thinking behind most of the guidance that parent would find.

While major media reporters hyperventilate about states that restrict or prohibit body altering drugs and surgeries for kids, it's rare that such news outlets report about how parents are losing the right to keep their children safe from trans ideology. Some states are either officially or unofficially cutting parents out of decisions to socially transition their children and even whether to give kids cross-sex hormones. In Maine, a sixteen-year-old can get cross-sex hormones without parental consent. Maine is also a "sanctuary" state that will not comply with warrants from other states related to transgender issues. Could a teen runaway who crosses state lines get hormones there? Almost certainly.

In Minnesota, a teen who has run away from home and is "managing [his or her] own financial affairs" can also manage his or her own medical and mental health care. Does that include cross-sex hormones? Almost certainly.

The answer to that question in California is certainly. Leave off the "almost." According to attorney Erin Friday, whose own trans ordeal you read about earlier, "We have a law that allows twelve-year-olds to leave their family home for any reason and go into a residential facility. And if that child goes into that residential facility and then becomes a dependent of the state at the age of twelve, that child can then dictate their own medical treatments."

In Washington state, if a child of *any* age runs away from home for the purpose of getting "gender-affirming care," the state will not return the child to his or her parents or let them know where their kid is.

About a dozen states considered politically blue have passed "sanctuary" laws for trans procedures. Details vary from state to state, but even where it's not official policy, "non-affirming" parents have had difficulty getting their children returned to them once they've crossed state lines.

Because teen girls make up the majority of those who suddenly present with confusion about their sex, boys can be overlooked. But they comprise about 30 percent of the total of afflicted teens. And the rise in claims of being the opposite sex among boys, while not as great as that of girls, is nevertheless astonishing.

Jamie Reed says that many boys who came to her clinic wanting to transition mentioned wanting to escape the "toxic masculinity" label. Telling boys, especially if they're white and heterosexual, that they're de facto "toxic" is typical in progressive and liberal schools that push a "social justice" agenda. Identifying as the opposite or no sex is often the only way for a boy to shed the label.

As with the girls, these boys often have multiple mental health and emotional issues. Many have suffered intense emotional upheaval, or are on the autism spectrum, have ADHD, OCD, or personality disorders.

Because the United States has no central database of its residents' medical histories, it's difficult to determine the number of boys afflicted. But other countries where mass trans indoctrination of kids is taking place do have central health record databases, and the figures from those give hints about the extent of the US problem.

In the United Kingdom, there was a 1,646 percent increase in boys referred to the central gender clinic between 2011 and 2022. In Spain, the increase in boys referred for treatment for gender confusion was 1,233 percent between 2013 and 2021. Sweden saw a 467 percent increase between 2013 and 2020.

The trans express has stations everywhere. So everywhere a troubled teen or preteen looks for a way to deal with angst, no matter what is causing it, he'll be dropped at the same destination.

Josie's son got cut from his sports team. It had been his whole life, his whole identity. Miserable, he found a new identity: as a girl.

Emily's son was gay, didn't want to be, and struggled with the stigma. "But he didn't want to work on that," says Emily. "I think he thought, 'If I become a woman, my attraction to men will be normal.'"

Kate, a school librarian, noticed that more kids were calling themselves trans but didn't think much about it until she went to a local women's group meeting. Of the ten women in the group, four had adolescent family members—children, nieces, nephew, grandkids—who claimed to be transgender. Four out of ten? How was that possible? The more she looked into the explosion in the numbers of kids claiming to be something they weren't, the more impossible it seemed.

Then her thirteen-year-old son told her that he was trans, too.

She searched for help. "Everywhere we went, the question was, 'What are your pronouns?'" She had no one to turn to. Reading the research, she discovered what medicalization would mean for her boy: a healthy body injured and his lifespan shortened. "Our kids have been betrayed."

These women poured out their painful stories about their sons in a September 2023 webinar sponsored by Parents With Inconvenient Truths About Trans, a support group for parents whose kids have rejected their sex. Groups like this one have sprung up in recent years on the internet, connecting parents who found themselves blindsided by sudden proclamations by sons and daughters who'd been seduced into the belief they're something other than sons and daughters.

Ellie* used to think that parents who didn't affirm their gender-confused kids were on the far-right fringe, or were misinformed, or fire-and-brimstone evangelicals—or all of the above. Definitely not enlightened liberals like herself. To the extent she thought of it at all, she'd have assumed that only conservatives questioned their kids wanting to "transition."

Then the cult came for her kid.

"I love John Stewart and John Oliver and Stephen Colbert," says Ellie. "And my son was right next to me watching these guys. And I didn't get it. I didn't get the damage that was being done. I don't think that they were wrong on everything. But I think what they created was a disaster everybody, for our kids, for the adults who don't see it, you know, to create such a polarizing environment, where people honestly believe that anybody who has an opposing viewpoint is either stupid or corrupt, is horrible."

The old Ellie would have counted anyone who warned against transgender ideology among those stupid, corrupt people until her fourteen-year-old son Carter* sent her and her husband Horst* a text that said: *I don't feel like a girl but I feel more like a girl than a boy.*

The year prior, 2019, Carter had attempted suicide by overdosing on his ADHD medicine. It had been apparent for some time that he was not doing well emotionally, and in 2020, adding to the stress of Covid lockdowns, remote school, and isolation, his mom was diagnosed with breast cancer. She'd begun chemo. That might have been Carter's tipping point.

And in a less chaotic time, despite her own indoctrination, Ellie might have questioned whether his pronouncement made any sense. Although he was no jock, Carter was a very masculine boy, attracted to girls, and with no earlier signs of a gender disorder. But when Carter insisted that his family call him by a new name and pronouns, and said he wasn't going to engage with anybody who didn't, Ellie and Horst offered no resistance.

"As I look back on it, I'm pretty amazed how primed for this we were because, already on NPR, they were already really pushing the stories of these transgender kids, normalizing it, making it seem like a medical condition," recalls Ellie. "So we knew that kids could go on medication. We knew that you had to affirm. It was crucial that you affirm. You know, the name and the pronoun were really important for their mental health. And so we said, 'Yeah, you know, of course we're going to call you by the new name and we're going to respect your pronouns.'"

Ellie consulted with the pediatrician who'd cared for Carter since he was born, a woman she thought of as a friend. The doctor quickly referred the family to a gender clinic. Ellie and Horst told the clinic's social worker they didn't want Carter on medication and the social worker said she understood. But immediately after the clinic visit, Carter started badgering his parents for puberty blockers. He wouldn't let up, screaming and crying and demanding. At first, Ellie held the line. But his behavior kept getting more extreme.

Carter had always worn his hair long. One day, on a dare from his new internet friends, he decided to chop it all off.

"I went for a walk and I came home to find him running barefoot in the street with his hair all hacked," says Ellie. "He looked like somebody from, you know, *One Flew Over the Cuckoo's Nest*. And I came in the house and there were piles of hair all over the house."

Ellie worried what he might do next.

In the back of her mind was Carter's earlier suicide attempt, and the constant drumbeat from media that children who aren't affirmed kill themselves. She and Horst asked the social worker for information on the blockers Carter had been demanding, hoping this medication might calm his increasing distress.

"She said, perfectly safe and reversible. You know, absolutely no side effects. You know, there's some concern about bone density problems, but that's all.'"

It didn't feel right, yet Ellie felt she had to agree.

"But the minute I consented to it, I just knew something was wrong," she says. "This was after my surgery where I could finally start to think straight again. I just felt like, this doesn't seem right. I started researching."

Meanwhile, Horst took Carter for his first shot. It would block the effects of puberty for the next three months.

Ellie had worked in public health for thirty years. Unlike the average parent, she knew how to search for and find relevant studies and she knew how to read them. Were these drugs truly "perfectly safe and reversible"? She needed to see the evidence for herself.

She read everything she could find. None of the available research supported the clinic social worker's assertions that puberty blockers were safe or reversible.

Now, truly worried, she asked the social worker: where's the data?

"She sent me this document, this email that had maybe fifty links in it. Every single one of them was very positive, nothing was mentioned about any controversy whatsoever. Nothing."

One of the links was to a document published by a respected university called "What We Know about Gender Affirming Care." It included dozens more links to research papers and articles. But none of those links led to any data showing puberty blockers were safe or reversible.

"I started looking at these things and seeing that none of them applied to this cohort. Some of them were completely irrelevant. And I thought, did the clinicians, like, did the social worker even read this stuff?"

Meanwhile, Carter's emotional state was worsening rather than improving on the blockers. He was angrier than before, more erratic, more oppositional. And now he was demanding cross-sex hormones.

When Ellie called with her concerns, the clinic suggested a team meeting.

"And they were very reassuring. '*Look, we're not going to move forward with hormones or anything. This a family decision. Nobody's going to push this on you. This is not going to happen.*' But then this one, they have a pediatric gynecologist at the meeting for my male child. And she says, 'Well, forty-one percent of these kids will commit suicide if they don't get affirmative care.'"

Having read and digested all the available research herself, Ellie knew that was false.

"And I let her have it. I said, '*You have no idea where those statistics come from, do you? Those statistics are lies. They're made up. They're based on garbage. And having a child who's already had a suicide attempt, I'm exceptionally offended by that.'* And she kind of backed down and apologized all over herself, but I figured it out then. These people didn't know what they were talking about."

She needed to get him off the blockers. Carter needed therapy, someone to help deal with his emotional issues. The clinic, though, would only refer Carter to gender-affirming therapists. With so many kids experiencing isolation and depression due to the Covid lockdowns, everyone else was booked.

Meanwhile, she tried to stall on Carter's next puberty blocker shot. Carter refused to go to school and was becoming more belligerent, screaming at people for "misgendering" him and demanding estrogen. Not knowing what else to do, and still a good liberal convinced that affirmation was the answer, Horst took him in to get another dose. The clinic was out of the three-month shots. They gave him one that would last six months.

Ellie was frantic. Reading the research, she'd discovered that blockers not only stopped visible bodily changes but also blocked the crucial brain development that occurs during puberty.

"It was devastating because I knew that this stuff wasn't safe and that he wasn't developing neurologically the skills that he needed. He wasn't developing critical thinking skills. He wasn't developing the capacity to understand long-term consequences. All the things that you would need to know to figure out whether or not this made any sense at all."

She called the clinic again, hoping she could persuade the clinical director to agree that Carter should be referred out to a non-affirming out-of-network therapist.

"And so she said, '*Well, the social worker did recommend your child start hormones. Did you know that?'* And I said, no, I didn't know that. I said, what criteria do you use to determine who will benefit and who won't? And she said, '*We don't really have criteria.*'"

No criteria? At all? Ellie couldn't believe her ears. She pointed out the risk that moving Carter from puberty blockers onto cross-sex hormones would render him sterile.

"She didn't seem to think the fertility was a big deal. '*Yeah, they do, but he'll get these nice curves and small breasts. He'll probably need implants because they won't really get that big. So probably need implants. But his skin will get softer.'* She said, *'It's not like testosterone for the girls. It's much gentler for the boys.'* I mean, this is insanity."

In the meantime, Carter had been emailing the endocrinologist, demanding a cross-sex hormone prescription. The endocrinologist responded that the team supported his decision to medically transition. But they couldn't legally get around his mother's refusal to consent.

Ellie was being pummeled from all sides, everyone trying to break down her resistance. Her husband was pressuring her to approve the cross-sex hormones. Her son was screaming at her and berating her. And the medical professionals were telling them that they were right and Ellie was wrong.

But Ellie stood firm.

She knew the claims that not affirming kids would lead them to suicide were false, but her son had attempted to kill himself before all this trans insanity began. So, for Carter, there was still a suicide risk, and it came from going along with this madness.

"I thought if he did this and he figured out that it was a lie he'd kill himself. He wouldn't survive that."

By 2022, Carter was no longer on puberty blockers and had been dismissed from the gender clinic as a patient without getting a cross-sex hormone prescription. Ellie discovered he was making appointments with his pediatrician without her approval. She hand-delivered a letter to the doctor, citing all the studies she'd read about the harms of cross-sex hormones and making it clear that she did not consent.

She also saw that Carter had pulled up a webpage on their home computer for do-it-yourself hormones.

"There were people called bathtub brewers. So these people buy raw materials from China and they make estrogen in their own homes and they sell it online," says Ellie. "I saw this page was open on the computer and I asked him about it and he said, *'I was looking at that for some friend.'"*

The red flags went up.

Mysterious lab documents arrived, showing that Carter had had blood tests to check his hormone levels.

When she confronted the doctor, she got denials. They'd just run some tests because his vitamin D levels were low, the doctor claimed.

Ellie checked Carter's texts and discovered messages back and forth with an older girl at school. The girl was eighteen and Carter was sixteen. She hadn't adopted a gender identity but was what a number of mothers of gender-confused boys call a cheerleader. These are girls who, quite literally, cheer boys on who show any signs of interest in transgenderism.

"They take them shopping for girl clothes, or they give them their girl clothes, and they really, you know, give the kids, the boys, a lot of attention. Now, adolescent boys, I mean, I don't know if you remember, but I certainly remember, the adolescent boys are so naïve when it comes to girls, and dating, and emotions, and sex. Girls are way ahead of the boys, and especially a child who has mental health issues and other issues and can't quite navigate the social landscape, to have this kind of attention from girls can be really exhilarating and confusing, I think. You know, here you finally get attention from girls, but they're telling you *you're* a girl too and they're giving you girls' clothes and they're giving you a lot of support to not be male."

The girl's parents were also committed to transgender ideology. They became Carter's "glitter family." Glitter moms, glitter dads, and glitter families are often trans ideologues, but are sometimes predators. They might be strangers, friends of the family, or extended family members. What they all have in common is their eagerness to act as stand-ins for a child's real parents when a mom and/or dad balks at a child assuming a trans identity. These glitter crews might do almost anything to undermine the parents' refusal to affirm. Some merely arrange for a kid to get a chest binder or a tuck kit (to hide the bulge of a penis) behind the parents' backs. Others actively campaign to get children to run away from home.

With her parents' full support and consent, Carter's school friend had bought bathtub hormones online. She then injected Carter with them. But, from his texts, Ellie could see that the girl had somehow messed up the injection. So Carter had turned to his pediatrician.

"[The pediatrician] instructed him on how to inject this street drug made by somebody in their home."

The blood tests that Ellie was told were simply to determine his vitamin D levels actually were designed to ascertain his baseline sex hormone levels so he would know how much of the illegally produced estrogen to inject into his body. The pediatrician planned to monitor his hormone levels as he continued this black market cross-sex treatment.

Ellie was stunned. She'd always considered Carter's pediatrician a friend. The woman had even come to visit her when she was in the hospital undergoing breast cancer treatment. And now, she was facilitating this deception. This doctor was coaching him on how to take drugs that, even if they were legally prescribed, could harm him irreparably. But bathtub hormones could be tainted with anything. The recklessness of the doctor's behavior bordered on criminal.

A complaint filed with the medical board went nowhere, but the bigger problem was the family supplying the drugs.

Ellie wanted to press charges but Carter was still fragile. Some of his texts and social media posts showed that he was still contemplating suicide. She worried he'd make another attempt if she got his friend and her parents in legal trouble.

She couldn't risk calling the cops. But she could use what she knew as leverage.

Carter refused to believe taking the bathtub hormones was illegal until Ellie read him the statutes. What they were doing could earn the glitter family as much as a year in prison and $1,000 fine.

"When he heard that, he fell apart. He was so terrified something would happen to this family and this girl. And I said, '*Here's the deal. Nothing will happen to them as long as nothing happens to you. And we're done with this. We're going to confiscate this medication. And you're not going to do anything. The minute something happens to you, it's over for them.*' And that's how I got him to stop the drugs."

But the danger for Carter isn't actually over.

He is now at college, more than 2,000 miles away from home. Ellie knows that it's possible for him to get cross-sex hormones if he's determined. She's resigned herself to the fact that she has no control over that. Her biggest fear now is genital surgery.

"Surgery will destroy him. Will destroy him. I've talked to enough detransitioners, male detransitioners, to know this. There's no real recovery from that."

By now, you might have noticed a pattern in these cases. It's not just preexisting mental health conditions that leave a kid vulnerable to trans ideology. You can trace almost every case to an emotional disturbance unrelated to transgenderism. For a great many kids, it was the unprecedented isolation and fear brought on by the Covid lockdowns. For Beth Bourne's daughter Elisa, it was a sexual attack on another child. The source of Carter's angst was his mother's breast cancer diagnosis. For Sophia, it appears to have been her father's pulling away from her when he remarried and started a new family.

Sophia was a quiet child. Homeschooled from second through fifth grade, she began attending a progressive independent school in Chicago from sixth grade on. Preferring to sit at home to playing in the park with friends, Sophia didn't quite fit in. "I remember going to parent-teacher conferences and the teacher said, you know, she does well academically, obviously," recalled her mom, Jeannette Cooper. "She's super smart and all that stuff. She has trouble kind of connecting with her peers."

As often happens when a kid doesn't fit in, Sophia was bullied mercilessly.

Still, as far as Jeannette knew, even if Sophia's tormentors at school sometimes made the kid's life hell, she seemed happy when the two of them were together.

Jeannette was what most kids would call a cool mom. Super-progressive, she eschewed rigid stereotypes. She wore her light brown hair punk style, short on one side and shaved on the other.

Sophia, by contrast, had lush, long dark wavy hair, and preferred more feminine styles.

Though her relationship with her mom was close and secure, the bond didn't appear quite so stable with her dad.

"I mean, a third of his custodial visits, which were about twenty-four hours in a week, a third of them he missed because he was out of town working," said Jeannette. "He's gone on some business trip. Yeah, so, yeah, out of, you know, fifty-two weeks in a year, he probably saw her about thirty."

Meanwhile, because Jeannette was working longer hours, the child was spending more time by herself.

Although Sophia had been getting less and less of her father's attention, she seemed to have genuine affection for her new stepmom, a licensed psychotherapist, and she adored her new baby half-sister.

In the summer of 2019, Sophia took a ten-day vacation with her dad and stepmom.

At seven thirty on the Sunday evening that Jeannette was due to pick her up, she sent her ex a text that she was on her way. Her ex wrote back that Sophia wanted to stay another night. Jeannette said no. That wasn't their agreement.

She drove the ten minutes to her ex-husband's house and texted again, saying she was outside and waiting.

This time, her ex didn't respond at all.

Another text was also ignored. She called on the phone.

"I don't remember whether he answers or not, but he comes outside. And I get out of my car and say, you know, 'Where's Sophia?'"

He told Jeannette that Sophia wasn't coming. Check with her to-morrow.

She begged her ex-husband to explain why her daughter didn't want to come home. All he would say is that Sophia would call.

"I got in the car and I actually wrote to my attorney at that moment, and I said something is wrong. I don't know what's happening right now, but something."

By the morning, Jeannette still hadn't heard anything. She willed herself to stay calm. This shouldn't have happened but it didn't neces-sarily mean anything. Sophia was about to turn thirteen. That's the age when kids start to rebel, she reminded herself. Even a sweet quiet kid like Sophia could do it.

"So then sometime in the afternoon, I saw an email pop up," said Jeannette.

It was from Sophia. In it, the child claimed she was trans and said, "I'm going to stay at dad's while you process this."

Jeannette didn't believe that Sophia had come up with that line her-self about processing the trans claim. She also didn't think for a minute that her kid was trans. She didn't believe anyone was trans—and she'd made that clear on many occasions with her daughter. She's spoken with Sophia about how transgenderism promotes worn-out sexual stereo-types. There was no "right" way to be a woman, Jeannette had explained to her daughter, and no need to pretend to be male if a woman didn't fit the conventional image of femininity. A woman can be anything she wants to be, dress however she chooses, live her life in whatever way she wants. She was still a woman.

Jeannette thought she'd succeeded in instilling these values in her daughter. But her daughter's email showed otherwise.

"I gave her a call later that night," says Jeannette. "And I said, 'Hey, you know, you have to come home.' And she said, she sounded so weird to me, a different person."

Sophia sounded angry and frustrated. She told Jeannette she was a bad mom who didn't care about her, who didn't really love her. Jeannette couldn't have known it at the time, but this is the script that trans activists use when they persuade kids to run away from home: that parents who don't agree with trans ideology are abusive and don't love them.

"I thought, what is happening? I don't know who I'm talking to right now. Like overnight, you are a different person."

Jeannette forced herself to remain calm, despite the untrue and hurtful things her child was saying. She listened quietly and then repeated: Sophia had to come home. Once she did, Jeannette reasoned, they'd work it out.

But Sophia didn't come home.

Meanwhile, her ex bought Sophia a new phone and tried to switch Sophia's account to it. Because the old phone was on Jeannette's mobile plan, he couldn't do it. But Jeannette could. She bought a new phone, and had Sophia's account transferred to it, "And then I opened up her iCloud and all of her messages. And I could see that [the stepmom] had helped this situation happen."

Sophia's stepmother had been playing glitter mom, actively encouraging the girl to leave her mother's home and pursue a trans identity, and offering whatever help the girl might need to do that. In her texts with the child, the stepmom strategized about how Sophia could move some of her belongings without her mother noticing.

Maybe Sophia's father wasn't giving her the attention he had when her parents lived together, but the child was getting positively love-bombed by her new glitter relative.

In one text, the stepmom wrote: *"I admire your courage. It would be great to talk at some point about what you want to be called. Ash? And any other stuff you want to shift. No hurry, but just know that I am open to any shifts you would like to make in name/pronoun/etc."*

In another, the glitter/stepmom wrote: *"I am still so surprised to hear about your mom's view on trans identity. It seems to me that she is questioning if she identifies as a woman . . ."*

In other words, by glitter mom's logic, the only reason Jeannette Cooper could possibly be skeptical of transgenderism was if she was harboring her own secret trans identity.

The text messages between the two also made it clear that Sophia's own therapist was coordinating with the stepmom about Sophia running away.

As for Sophia, once she adopted her new identity, the greatest rival for her dad's attention became her greatest ally. And at the school where she had never fit in? Sophia was an instant rock star.

"[The school] said to me that, oh, this was going to give them such an opportunity to learn so much," recalls Jeannette. "They were so happy to celebrate their first trans student. They sent out emails to all the parents in the entire school to announce their first trans student."

Jeannette's lawyer filed an emergency petition with the court. It seemed to be a straightforward situation. Sophia had been living with Jeannette since the divorce and this was the first time anyone questioned the custody agreement.

The lawyers squabbled about Sophia's trans claim. And then the judge asked whether Sophia had ever expressed a desire to commit suicide.

As it turned out, after the divorce, when Sophia was nine years old, she had said something vague, like, "*I wish I weren't alive.*"

Sophia had never threatened to actually harm herself but that was all it took. Like most people, the judge was aware of the claim that kids who said they were trans would commit suicide if not affirmed. Like most people, the judge had no idea the claim was false.

She ordered Sophia to remain with her father.

Jeannette has only seen her daughter twice since then: once in family therapy and once, three years later, for a visit in a coffee shop that her ex arranged. But she has followed Sophia on social media. The girl is now a beautiful young woman. She dresses in feminine styles. She currently appears to be calling herself non-binary. That can serve as an in-between identity. Kids often start calling themselves non-binary before going full trans; they also often claim to be non-binary when they're on the way out of the cult but not quite ready to make a full break.

Jeannette, heartbroken, waits for the day when she'll get to see her daughter again. She knows it will happen. She just doesn't know when. She doesn't blame Sophia. Her daughter was a child. It's the adults who facilitated their estrangement.

No matter how many tens of thousands of children are afflicted by this madness, the worst of the insanity always can be traced back to the adults—the ones who should know better, but never do.

Chapter 7

Is Transgender Actually a Thing (and Is It Just One Thing)?

"It's all make believe, isn't it?"

—Marilyn Monroe

If you live in or near a progressive city, you've probably run into a number of men in skirts. They're pushing their cart in front of you on the supermarket checkout line, or sitting at the table next to you in that nice Thai restaurant, or directing you to the plumbing section at Home Depot. But no matter how much time they spend perfecting their makeup techniques or blow-drying their long locks, you almost always clock them as guys. And it's always sort of sad. I know just one guy who identifies as a woman who passes well—at least, when you look at him. But when you hear his voice, you know it's a man talking.

Testosterone has more dramatic external effects on a woman than estrogen has on a man. A woman on testosterone will start losing her hair, just like her dad did. The cross-sex hormone will allow her to grow a beard—lots of body hair, too. It will cause her voice to drop from a soprano to a tenor range. While a man who takes estrogen usually just looks and sounds like a guy in drag, a woman on testosterone can often pass as a man.

That was certainly true of Claire* when I met her. A pleasant looking, stocky young person with a bit of a beard, arms covered in tattoos, whose sandy hair was beginning to recede, she fooled me at first, when we met in person. Later, we spent a long time on a Zoom call and I learned her full story. The first thing she said that made me sit up and take notice was that she'd never actually felt that she was a man. I wanted to know more. Why would anyone who thought of herself as female put herself through all that she'd been through?

"I knew I was biologically female, but yeah, I did think that it would make things easier," says Claire. "I did think I would be more respected, taken seriously, just be safer out in the world physically. I wouldn't have to deal with any homophobia, any external homophobia or even internal homophobia."

Claire is bisexual and comes from a fairly conservative family. She worried family members would reject her if they learned she wasn't entirely straight, but didn't seem to think she'd have the same problems if she "transitioned" to living as if she were the opposite sex.

"My first exposure to the whole transgender thing was I took a Women and Gender Studies class at my college," she told me. "And the last two days were all about transgender people."

The year was 2015. The teacher played the Jazz Jennings documentary for the class. Claire was riveted.

Back in her room, she fired up her laptop, began Googling, and immediately came across images of Aydian Dowling, who was born a woman but now identified as a man. Aydian was a body builder, and looked it: short beard, moustache, muscular chest, bulging biceps, broad shoulders—everything about her screamed "male." The only hint that she was actually a woman were her mastectomy scars, but those were partly covered by wisps of dark chest hair. Anyone who didn't recognize the telltale scarring for what it was would have taken her for the most macho of men.

"I identified with it so much that it, like, scared me. I remember that I just like closed my laptop. Yeah, because I was like, this is too much."

But she kept going back online, finding more and more people who had "transitioned" and were raving about the results on Youtube. They all claimed to be so happy.

Until earlier that year, the medical standards of care had called for three months of therapy prior to getting a cross-sex hormone prescription. But, due to activists' pressure campaign, the standards had just changed. Now, nothing more was required than "informed consent." All guard rails were removed. And because Claire was over eighteen, she didn't need her parents' approval to begin taking testosterone. Insurance covered everything except for about a ten-dollar monthly co-pay. It was almost too easy.

The male hormone flooding through her system supercharged her libido. She'd always been shy around men. Testosterone changed that.

"Like growing up in high school, I had a few boyfriends and I just didn't like how they would treat me, like a woman, or would sexualize me. I don't know. I just didn't like it. But when I was passing as male I felt like I could be as masculine as I wanted and they would still accept me."

She hooked up with several different men. "They were always my friends first because I wanted to be, like, safe. I didn't want to just, like, go into a scary situation."

After watching Youtube videos of women who'd had "top surgery" and claimed to be ecstatic at the changes, Claire signed up to get a double mastectomy.

"You'll see those kind of top surgery reveal videos where you see them for the first time out of surgery and they get to look down at their own chest for the first time And they start crying because they're so happy."

So, that's what Claire was expecting.

But the reality was different. Somewhere in the back of her mind, she'd half imagined her chest would resemble Aydian Dowling's. Hers was simply flat. She had nothing to celebrate; all she felt was shock.

It didn't deter her.

By 2018, she was out of school, working full-time in the service industry, and going by the name Max*. She'd grown a beard. Everyone at work just assumed she was a guy, including a rather striking young woman with long dark hair named Rhonda* who worked in a different department.

Claire, now Max, felt an immediate attraction to Rhonda but didn't see how she could act on it. There was some irony to this. Claire had done all she could to present herself as a man because she hoped for more acceptance. But now, she was afraid that this charming co-worker would reject her if she knew the truth about "Max." So, they'd go out in a group after work to a bar, but she kept a bit of distance. This went on for almost a year. Then Rhonda told "Max" she was attracted to "him" and Claire was in a bind.

"I decided to, like, come out to her because I didn't see a way out of it at that point," Claire recalls. "I said something along the lines of, I'm afraid you won't like me anymore after I tell you this. And you know, she's pretty open. So she was like, no, it's okay. Tell me. And then I said, 'I'm trans.' And I remember her saying that it doesn't *not* matter, but it doesn't matter enough for her feelings to change about me. So yeah, I mean, it was great to feel that sort of acceptance where I could, like, let her into a big part of my life that I previously couldn't."

But Rhonda "identified" as straight. She'd never before been attracted to a biological female. Claire figured that that meant Rhonda was attracted to male genitalia and masculinity and to some extent, that made Claire put more pressure on herself.

"I didn't feel like there was any pressure coming from her whatsoever. But for me, yeah, I think I had this expectation that I've put on myself to be like the manliest man, you know?"

Claire decided she had to get phalloplasty. She actually said she'd rather die than *not* get phalloplasty. "That's really how I felt. But I was scared at the same time. It was a lot of different emotions. It was hope. It was being nervous and terrified. It was being excited. It was fear of the unknown. It was all these things at the same time. But yeah, I did feel like I needed to try because I had become, I think, so dead set that this was almost like my purpose. Like transition was my purpose."

Only then, she thought, would she feel good about herself and be able to start her life.

According to therapist Stephanie Winn, thoughts like these aren't uncommon among those chasing the transgender dream, and are very much like those of girls who have eating disorders. Young people become obsessed with the erroneous idea that happiness awaits once their bodies are sufficiently altered. The term that applies is "body dysmorphia," which, though it sounds similar to "dysphoria," means something different. It's a persistent belief that something about the body is the source of their emotional problems and by "fixing" the body, their problems will be solved.

"I've noticed a lot of similarities between the sort of thought patterns associated with gender dysphoria, body dysmorphia, and eating disorders, with obsessive-compulsive disorder," says Winn. "It gets channeled into this fixation on 'my body' or 'my gender' or 'my gender identity' or what have you, that must be a problem. And then you have this whole kind of set of behaviors, the compulsions that develop around this."

Claire knew that other young women had suffered debilitating complications as a result of what's euphemistically called "bottom surgery." Yet she became certain that the reward would be worth the cost, whatever that cost turned out to be.

It would take numerous surgeries to reach her goal.

First came the hysterectomy and metoidioplasty (enlarging the clitoris). Surgeons closed her vaginal opening, removed her uterus and fallopian tubes, but left one ovary at her request. They cut the little tendon that connects the clitoris to the rest of the body. "After I had recovered from that surgery, they put my urethra through my clitoris. So I could like pee through the clitoris and it was kind of like a little bit higher than it would be on a biological female."

Before surgeons could complete the phalloplasty itself, they needed "donor" flesh to create the penis facsimile.

That turned out to be the most disabling procedure of all.

"For the phalloplasty, I took my donor site off of my right thigh," she recalls. "And that was probably the hardest part about recovering, not even like, you know, that they messed around down there and moved stuff around and attached stuff. It was my thigh."

She hadn't realized that removing a piece of her thigh would make it so weak. She couldn't lift it or bend it for months.

"So I would literally have to go to the bathroom standing up, which you can imagine is, like, very difficult. Because you can't bend your hip. So, like, I would have to be leaning back diagonally trying to go to the bathroom."

Through it all, she had been hearing horror stories from other women who'd been through phalloplasty. And almost everyone had complications, those she saw on Youtube and those she spoke to in person.

"So one is, if you don't get all of the body hair, you know, lasered off before they create your urethra, you'll basically get chronic UTIs because all the bacteria will like stick onto the hair inside of your urethra. And so I know [women] who, every few months, they need to go to the doctor and they'll put something up their dick and strip out all the hair from inside their urethra and pull it out. Yeah, like, that sounds horrible."

But the women said they'd do it all over again. It made Claire think that this had to be the most amazing experience because of what they had gone through to get where they were.

Another woman told her about getting strictures. That's when the body reacts as if the neo-urethra is an open wound that needs to close up and heal. So, it would close. And it would scar. The woman had to use a device similar to a knitting needle to keep it open. Every day, she'd stick this device into her urethra to keep it from closing. It was painful. It was traumatic. Yet, she too, said it was worth it.

"I thought about it like, this is like the fight of my life. Like, I need to get through this so that I can be happy."

At the end of many months' torment, she had a facsimile penis.

But it wasn't a functioning organ. It was incapable of an erection or penetrative sex. Still, it felt to her as if "mission accomplished." She experienced that gender euphoria that all those other women had raved about.

At least, for a while she did.

"I was like so excited that I had a bulge in my pants. I was like, oh, yeah, I finally get to fill out my boxer briefs."

But as time passed, the euphoria faded. And she began to rethink.

"I spent so much time, you know, obsessing about this. And I finally reached my goal. And now what?"

Claire was one of the lucky ones. Though her surgical ordeal was long, painful, and altogether brutal, she didn't suffer any of the complications she'd been told about. Still, she'd started developing health problems due to being on testosterone for a number of years.

"My cholesterol was going up. And, like, my triglycerides and stuff. And that's something that I've heard happens with trans guys and also gaining weight. I've gained weight. I think my ideal weight is somewhere around 150 pounds. But I got up to like 180."

The psychological effects also began weighing heavily on her.

"I feel like transition kind of gave me the promise of an easier life, a better life, a happier life, and being more authentic. And my experience has kind of led me to be, like, I don't feel like I'm being authentic. Because I feel like people assume that I grew up male and all this stuff."

By the time we met, Claire had been off testosterone for several months. At first, she told herself she would stop taking it simply because she wanted to reverse some of the health problems it had caused. She hadn't yet faced the possibility of detransitioning. But slowly, she's figured out that that might be the way she's heading.

According to the Society for Evidence-Based Gender Medicine (SEGM), the average time from transgender surgery to regret is about eight years. Claire started the process in 2015. We spoke in mid-2023. The timeline fits.

"I know that when I did find people that were also detransitioning, it was like they were saying things that I had been thinking, but I had never heard another person say," says Claire. "Everyone talks about transition as if it's all sunshine and rainbows. But these [detransitioners] were saying very real things that I had also experienced and felt."

Now that she's no longer on cross-sex hormones, her skin is clearing up and feels softer. The hair she's lost won't ever grow back, but at least her hair has stopped falling out. She's started experiencing emotions that she hadn't felt for years, because testosterone tends to dull the highs and lows.

But what if she wanted to go all the way back—or as far as it's possible for her to go at this point?

"That's the tough thing, is that if I decide to have surgeries in the other direction, detransitioning, it's going to be a lot harder because right now there's no, like, I wouldn't get insurance coverage."

Due to trans activism, insurers in a number of states are required to cover all the procedures and drugs that allow someone to mimic the opposite sex as "medically necessary" care. As of this writing, there's no insurance coverage for detransition care anywhere in the United States.

"[What] I would ideally like to do is get a hair transplant. In an ideal world, I would get my hairline back to normal. I would probably get some kind of feminization voice surgery so that my voice goes back up to sounding like a female. I would get breast reconstruction." But her wish list includes some procedures that are simply not possible, not even with the best insurance.

"It would be cool to just, like, take my phallus and put it back on my thigh and my, now my thigh is normal."

Her thigh is permanently weakened. Her vagina is damaged beyond repair. Her reproductive system, other than one ovary, is gone.

None of that can be reversed.

"I kind of feel like, all right, I've learned my lesson. I appreciate womanhood now and I understand gender roles and their functionality and how they are important. And I have greater empathy than before for males and the expectations that are put on them. And I wish I could just like snap my fingers and go back in time, but keep those lessons with me. But I can't. That's not how life works."

Trans activists will tell you that people who regret their decisions and want to turn back the clock are rare. But how could anyone really know? It's easy to get cross-sex hormones and surgeries. Undoing the damage is mostly impossible. And if people are paying out of pocket to get surgeries to repair at least some of what's been done to them in the name of "gender-affirming care," no one is keeping records of it.

The World Health Organization promulgates what it calls International Classification of Diseases (ICD) codes for virtually everything a person might ask a doctor to treat. There are, as you'd imagine, codes for heart attack, stroke, and every type of cancer. There's a code for treatment for a rabbit bite. There are separate codes for a stubbed toe; one if the nail is damaged and another if it isn't. There are codes for every phase and type of "gender-affirming care."

There are no codes for detransition care. None.

If a doctor were to treat Claire in an attempt to mitigate some of what's been done to her body, it's anyone's guess how it would be noted on a chart. Cosmetic surgery? Probably. Given how much input trans activists have had on everything from media coverage to government regulations to medicine, it's reasonable to assume that's by design. If you can't code it, no one who searches for it will find it. If you can't find it, detransition care doesn't exist—and neither do detransitioners.

How many thousands of young people who bought into the promise of a better life in the past few years are still in the "honeymoon phase" of their trans adventure?

How many others will soon be in Claire's position, wishing they could take it all back?

Like Claire, for a lot of kids, their first exposure to trans indoctrination comes in college. A survey found almost 6 percent of college students claimed trans or non-binary identities.

Living apart from their families for the first time, in an environment where gender confusion is treated like a badge of honor, college kids are uniquely vulnerable as they try to fit in. They also have the freedom for the first time to make adult choices. But though they might legally be adults, they don't always have the emotional maturity to understand the lifelong ramifications of some of their choices. In the more progressive colleges and universities, virtually round-the-clock trans indoctrination is the norm.

Once college kids start imagining their bodies need altering, schools' insurers are often only too happy to cover the cost.

At least 150 colleges' health insurance policies cover amputating a girl's healthy breasts; surgically removing her uterus, ovaries, and genitals; and surgically constructing, from pieces sliced from her now irreparably damaged arm or thigh, a nonfunctioning replica of a phallus. Boys can get coverage for the removal of their testicles and scrotum, and inversion of their penises into the likeness of female genitals that might or might not function.

Some schools' insurance policies—another twenty-eight at last count—cover only cross-sex hormones.

Parents might be thousands of miles away. Those parents often don't find out that their legally adult but still immature offspring have changed names, started on cross-sex hormones, and scheduled surgeries until months later, when their college student comes home on vacation.

Those who live in red states or in less urban areas where trans ideology isn't promoted in schools can't assume their kids are safe. Laws against cross-sex hormones, puberty blockers, and unnecessary surgeries for minors are a start, and can protect the youngest. But laws leave anyone eighteen or older unprotected.

It should be apparent that there are countless reasons why kids and young adults become susceptible to transgender ideology. And none has anything to do with the fiction of having been born in the wrong body.

But some of the most visible "trans" people are older men who have lived as typical males for the first three, four, five, or even six decades of their lives, and now want to be called women. What gives?

Most people assume that, were they not cross-dressing full-time, such men would have simply been flamboyantly effeminate gay men.

That's a misconception. In a joint article, two prominent psychologists who study gender identity disorders, J. Michael Bailey, PhD, and Ray Blanchard, PhD, estimated that only about 25 percent of the males who identify as trans today are same-sex attracted.

The other approximately 75 percent—the vast majority—are heterosexual. These men often appear hyper-masculine before "coming out." They are more likely to be jocks than fashion designers. Think Bruce Jenner, the college running back and Olympic decathlon champion who adopted the name Caitlyn in 2015 and began appearing in women's clothing, makeup, and wigs. Before assuming a trans identity, such men typically get married, father children (Jenner fathered six by three wives), and have high-powered careers in male-dominated professions.

Then one day, seemingly out of the blue, they claim to be female, often insisting that they are lesbians—though obviously, a male lesbian is a contradiction in terms. Just as often, they demand immediate access to everything set aside for actual females, including their intimate spaces.

Because they begin cross-dressing due to sexual compulsion, straight male cross-dressers are a class apart, completely distinct from others with gender confusion, such as the adolescents and young adults you met in earlier chapters. They have almost nothing in common with gay male cross-dressers, except women's wear. Although gay men may also claim transgender identities, they'll typically do so as a continuation of a childhood gender disorder that begins as early as age two or three.

Though the first incidence of cross-dressing in straight males can begin around puberty, that's later than kids with childhood-onset.

The two main broad categories of heterosexual cross-dressing males are autogynephiles and transvestic fetishists. Though some experts believe they are two branches of the same disorder, they're actually distinct from one another, according to the published research.

That's important to know because the research shows that transvestic fetishists are more likely to engage in harmful deviant behavior toward others than autogynephiles. Transvestic fetishists are also less likely to surgically "transition," probably because they're less likely to have actual gender identity disorders. They're not typically confused or distressed about their sex; they know they are males.

But before we get much further, you're probably wondering: what on Earth is an autogynephile?

Blanchard, perhaps the most prominent researcher in the world when it comes to adult male gender identity disorders, coined the terms autogynephile and autogynephilia. The latter means love of (and lust for) oneself as a woman.

Autogynephilia is technically not a fetish but a paraphilia, which is an umbrella term used for aberrant sexual behavior. Just as all poodles are dogs but not all dogs are poodles, all fetishes are paraphilias but not all paraphilias are fetishes. Men with fetishes (and fetishes almost exclusively affect men) are sexually aroused by physical objects. The autogynephile, by contrast, is aroused by a fantasy involving his own body as the object of his lust. In a masturbatory reverie, an autogynephile imagines himself to either be a woman, or to have female body parts, such as a vagina and breasts. Though cross-dressing adds to that fantasy, the clothes and makeup are secondary. The fantasy of becoming a woman is the main event. And autogynephiles (sometimes abbreviated as AGPs) aren't drag queens, either. Drag queens are gay men who wear elaborate feminine costumes, often with an over-the-top burlesque esthetic. AGPs are more likely to emulate their wives, or whoever symbolizes their ideal woman fantasy.

A man with autogynephilia who once identified as transgender but no longer does, explained in a post on X what the experience was like for him:

> *AGPs will look in the mirror and see another person in the mirror ("there's this girl") that they fall in love with . . . this often becomes obsessive and devolves into an elaborate masturbatory life focused on this internal attraction to the narratized self projected on the mirror image.*

Between 80 and 90 percent of AGPs are sexually attracted to women, with the rest claiming a lack of attraction to *any* bodies but their own. It's not a stretch to assume that an autogynephilic male was the inspiration for the ancient Greek myth of Narcissus. In that tale, Narcissus becomes so enamored of his own image, mirrored in a pool of water, that he can do nothing but stare in adoration.

Joseph Burgo, PhD, a psychologist who treats men with the condition, believes many are subconsciously looking for a way out of the burdens of manhood. They find solace in what they imagine is the simpler existence of a woman.

The second major group of cross-dressing straight men that researchers have studied are the transvestic fetishists. The name of the disorder makes it easier to understand their compulsion. While it's also an aberrant sexual drive that also involves wearing female clothing, unlike autogynephiles, transvestic fetishists don't typically fantasize about having women's bodies or body parts when they masturbate. The clothes themselves deliver the sexual arousal and release. Some such men favor very specific garments and fabrics, which is the essence of fetishism.

The word fetish comes from *feitiço*, a Portuguese term that refers to a magical amulet or talisman. No doubt, men with transvestic fetishism consider the garments they wear to have something akin to magic, especially those who can't achieve orgasm without them.

Mental health professionals don't always agree whether transvestic fetishism should be labeled a fetish or should fall under the umbrella term paraphilia. But most of us aren't in a position where we need to come up with a clinical diagnosis. Since there's no way to determine a man's sexual disorder just by looking at him, it's probably safest to assume the guy making a show of using the toilet stall next to you or your daughter has a fetish.

There are several reasons I say this:

- The word "fetish" is immediately familiar to virtually everyone;
- It's an accurate dictionary term for sexual fixations on physical objects such as clothing;
- Although the DSM, as of today, lists transvestic fetishism under the umbrella "paraphilia" category, DSM categories and diagnostic criteria can and do change;
- The word alerts others that the man it describes might not be as

harmless and vulnerable as activists and our major media portray him to be.

The peer-reviewed papers about transvestic fetishists are scant, but reading them reveals these guys can sometimes exhibit dark compulsions.

A 2005 study conducted in Sweden found that 36 percent of transvestic fetishists said they'd committed acts of exhibitionism, and almost 14 percent said they were sexually turned on by pain. The paper also pointed to earlier research that showed as many as 20 percent of transvestic fetishists admitted to sexually molesting children.

This is just what they admitted to. Researchers who study sexually aberrant behavior have found that cross-dressing straight males can be deceptive when questioned about what they think, feel, and do.

It also should be noted: the online magazine *Reduxx* has been reporting for several years now about cross-dressing men getting arrested for committing sex crimes against children, engaging in exhibitionism, and other sexual offenses. Interestingly, although such crimes are typically covered in small local media in the places where they occur, they're almost entirely ignored by larger media outlets.

In earlier decades, most of these guys would have hidden their proclivities out of shame and fear of stigma, cross-dressing in secret, but otherwise leading the perfectly ordinary lives of perfectly ordinary husbands and fathers.

Today, AGPs and transvestic fetishists are getting "woman of the year" and other awards that were meant for females. They're cheered for their "courage" by an ideologically captured society that mostly has no idea what it's cheering.

For AGPs and transvestic fetishists in today's world, it's like Christmas every day.

Take, for example, the Spanish actor Juan Carlos Gascón who had, at best, a marginal film career until he was in his late forties. At that point, he renamed himself Karla Sofia Gascón and got cosmetic surgery to make himself appear less masculine. Not long after, at the age of fifty-two, he got his first big break playing a drug lord who goes through surgical transition in the film *Emilia Pérez*, for which he received a number of "best actress" nominations and awards, including a nomination as "best actress" from the Oscars.

Another man past middle age who almost no one had ever heard of before, Andrew (now Harper) Steele, became an instant sensation in the documentary *Will and Harper* for telling his friend, comedian Will Ferrell, he'd begun identifying as a woman, and taking a road trip with the actor while cross-dressing.

Think about the people who have become the faces of trans inclusivity, and who are featured in the news. Although socially induced gender confusion affects mostly teen girls, it's not girls' or women's faces we see when media looks for a spokesperson. We see, instead, older men dressed as women: Bruce/Caitlyn Jenner; Mark/Marci Bowers; Richard/Rachel Levine; Martin/Martine Rothblatt.

Not all straight male cross-dressers are activists, but those who are can be quite aggressive toward anyone who rejects their "identities" as real. Dr. Burgo has written that such rejection might be perceived by such a man as persecution, and even a threat to his very existence.

"His envy of biological women—for embodying the idealized state he longs for but can never truly reach—may lead to vindictive and physical assaults upon their persons. He wants to destroy them and the truth they embody."

Burgo also noted that such humiliation can be sexually arousing for autogynephilic males.

Blanchard has noted another peculiarity in AGPs that highlights the strangeness of this affliction, without necessarily increasing our understanding of it: " . . . in later years . . . autogynephilic sexual arousal may diminish or disappear, while the transsexual wish remains or grows even stronger."

Trans activists have expressed outrage that Blanchard called autogynephilia what it was. There's been a sustained public relations effort to uncouple straight male trans "identities" from the anomalous sexual compulsions that motivate them. But as a renowned expert on paraphilic disorders, and part of the working group for the *DSM-5*, the psychiatric manual that laid out the diagnostic criteria for this set of mental disorders, Blanchard can't easily be dismissed.

The psychologist also says that the ideological position isn't logical.

"Well, there is a disorder involved," he says. "And leaving aside reality, which is easy to do with the world of gender, if there's no disorder, then there's no third-party payment for any of these medical procedures."

Though the cross-dressing and fantasies start out in private, the compulsion gets stronger as the years go by, says Blanchard. "In some cases, the children are now grown, they've left the house. You know, the only one left to be harmed is the wife."

Until everything blew up, Becca* considered herself happily married. Sure, all marriages have their ups and downs, and Larry* had some strange quirks. But they'd enjoyed each other's company since they met in college.

He was smart, handsome, and a good provider, moving up with his company to regional sales manager within a year of their marriage.

Her first hint that something wasn't quite right came right around the time of his job promotion. Returning home from a business trip, he seemed exhausted, so Becca unpacked his suitcase for him. She tossed his laundry in the hamper, and hung his shirts and slacks in the closet.

She felt the slinky fabric before she saw it, something completely out of place at the bottom of a man's suitcase: a pair of blue satin panties. What on Earth?

The underwear were her own. So he wasn't cheating on her. Why did he take her undies to Tucson?

Larry laughed when she confronted him, *"I missed you, so I brought something along to remind me of you."*

Becca accepted his explanation but other incidents weren't as easy to dismiss. He'd begun shaving his chest and under his arms, claiming he did it because it was more hygienic and it kept him from sweating so much, which, he said, could create a problem at work where he had to look cool and in charge. But there was no simple explanation for the used makeup wipes in the bathroom wastebasket with what appeared to be blue eye shadow smeared on them. Becca was the only woman living in the house and hadn't worn blue eye shadow since her teens.

And in bed one night, Larry suggested they pretend that they were lesbians. "He wanted us both to dress in lingerie," recalls Becca.

That might have been a turn-on for her husband but for Becca, it was the ultimate turn-off. She told him, absolutely not.

The year was 2005. Bruce Jenner had not yet started calling himself Caitlyn. Becca had no idea what an AGP was or even that such men existed. She'd later learn that for men with the fetishistic disorder, this sort of sexual request was typical.

What she did know was that his behavior was becoming increasingly odd, enough so that she briefly considered divorce. Then, she got pregnant. She stayed.

Their baby was born prematurely. Becca had planned to return to work once their boy was about six months old, but the little one had breathing problems and anemia, and was hooked up to an IV in the neonatal ICU. Frantic with worry, Becca couldn't imagine delegating this fragile infant's needs to daycare workers. She felt she had no choice but to quit her job and take care of her son full-time.

She and Larry were sitting together in the chilly hospital waiting room, fluorescent lights flickering above their heads, oblivious to everything except concerns about their new little son. At least, that was Becca's frame of mind. Larry's mind was elsewhere. While they awaited word from the doctor, Larry took the opportunity to make a confession: he had been cross-dressing. He'd done it off and on since he was a teen, he said, stealing his mom's and his sister's underwear and other garments. It didn't mean he was gay, he assured her. He was as heterosexual as ever. But imagining himself as a woman sometimes helped to dissipate the constant stress that came from climbing the corporate ladder.

Becca was stunned. And yet, it made a kind of weird sense when she thought of all the earlier unexplained incidents. Still, with a sick baby to worry about, she couldn't focus on him or his issues. They'd need to go to marriage counseling, she said. Then she ended the conversation and put it out of her thoughts, to the extent possible.

Much later, she'd learn, when comparing notes with other women married to AGPs, that her situation was not unique. "They wait until the birth of the first baby. They wait until the woman is in a position where it's more difficult to leave."

And if that was his plan to hang onto her, it was a smart move because at that moment, she felt trapped.

In the back of her mind, she assumed a marriage counselor would tell Larry that what he was doing was damaging their marriage and if he wanted to save it, he'd have to stop.

"I could envision in some things there's compromise, but for this, it felt similar to infidelity to me," Becca recalls.

The counselor surprised Becca with her suggestions for what she called a "compromise": let Larry continue his cross-dressing but keep it to himself. He could rent a post office box where he could have catalogs for women's clothing and lingerie delivered. He could also have brochures mailed to him with information about retreats where men dress up as women together.

"That was the first I've ever heard of such a thing, but it sounded like, okay, not a really good idea." It certainly didn't sound like a compromise, since she'd be the only one compromising.

Becca stood firm: if he didn't stop the cross-dressing, she would leave him. Larry didn't want to lose her. He agreed. And things got back to normal. Mostly.

But their sex life began to suffer. Larry just didn't seem to be terribly interested in intimacy any more. Was it me, Becca wondered? "I always thought it was my fault. And what could I do better?"

Larry assured her that the problem was all his, a side effect of the medication his doctor had prescribed for his obsessive-compulsive disorder. She didn't question his explanation, especially since she'd noticed other side effects, including overall weight gain, and a rather off-putting increase in the fat on his chest. Poor Larry was developing man-boobs.

Still, somehow, despite the fact that they rarely had sex any more, she became pregnant again.

Their little boy was four years old and though he still had health problems, he was growing stronger. Larry made a bizarre comment that, maybe, he could help out if things got overwhelming for her by sharing breastfeeding responsibilities for the new baby.

Was he joking? He had to be. Becca brushed off his comment as a self-deprecating jab at how his OCD meds had redistributed his body fat. Years later, she'd learn that AGPs often fetishize breastfeeding—and that there was a better explanation for his development of man-boobs. Yes, it was caused by medication but it wasn't a side effect. It was the drug's intended effect. And the drug he was taking had nothing to do with treating his OCD.

By 2018, the trans craze was in full swing. Their once sickly son was eleven, healthy and robust. Their daughter, seven, had started first grade. Larry was out of town on another of his business trips. And Becca's minivan wouldn't start.

She didn't know where Larry left his car keys but she had to drive the kids to school and get to work. Searching his desk drawer in his home office, she found the keys to his Lexus, and something else: a vial of clear liquid and a box of syringes. The label listed the vial's contents: estradiol valerate. Estrogen.

Larry was taking estrogen.

After dropping the kids at school, she popped the trunk and found a stash of women's clothes, including some of her own that were supposed to have gone to Goodwill months before. He might have simply forgotten to drop off her old garments, but there were also several newer oversized nighties from Victoria's Secret and other high-end lingerie that he'd apparently bought for himself.

She called in sick to work and powered up the computer. It took a few tries but she was able to guess his email password pretty quickly.

Within hours, she knew everything, or almost everything. He'd been seeing another woman. On the nights he'd claimed he was playing tennis or poker, he was actually with her. He'd been taking estrogen on and off for years, since before her last pregnancy. That was what had dampened his sex drive and given him boobs. "And in those messages with the person he was having the affair with, she was all into the cross-dressing and feminizing him."

Their divorce freed Larry to cross-dress full-time. Pretty soon, he wasn't calling it cross-dressing any more. He wanted people to see him as a woman. He wanted the kids to call him "mom." Within earshot of his mortified children, he told people that he'd given birth to them.

"So they went through a lot of heartbreaking situations," recalls Becca. "As much as they wanted him to show up to things, it was embarrassing if he did, because people would ask all kinds of questions. And you don't want the other kids in school, like, seeing your dad, who's obviously not a woman, but is trying to look like a woman."

Larry's behavior was particularly painful for their son. Warming up for baseball games, other fathers would pitch balls to their kids. If Larry showed up at all, it was in heels and makeup.

"And [their son] would just pretend he had a headache and put his head down and cry because he was so embarrassed and so sad that he didn't have his dad there anymore who he looked up to," says Becca. "Larry was his hero when he was young, but every time he saw him, he would [not only] change more and more physically, but also changed his personality more."

Both children were distraught enough to need intensive therapy, but outwardly, at least, her daughter didn't seem quite so devastated as her son.

"She just said, 'He's trying to be you, mom.'"

And her daughter's observation appeared to be accurate. Becca and Larry both had brown hair, but after their split, Becca became a blonde. Soon, Larry went blonde, too, styling his hair in Becca's mid-length bob, despite his slightly receding hairline.

He had cosmetic surgery to feminize his face, and that, too, made him resemble Becca more. She doesn't believe it was coincidental. "He's totally trying to have my nose."

What's allowed Becca to stay strong is support from an online network of other wives whose cross-dressing husbands decided to "transition." They call themselves "trans widows," even though their husbands are still alive and some have stayed married to the men who now pretend to be women.

Those who've never gone through the trauma of having a husband and father decide he no longer wants to be a man can't begin to understand what the family goes through, Becca says.

"They're just in survival mode and they cannot even imagine a way out. They need support. They need support by their family, from their friends, from their church, and their community, just like a woman who's been in a battered relationship. Because mentally, that's where they are."

It should be apparent by now that there's nothing much to connect members of the different groups claiming trans status other than that they're all celebrated by believers in the ideology. A prepubescent child who is confused about his sex has almost nothing in common—symptom-wise or disorder trajectory-wise—with a grown man who furtively dresses up in his wife's undies while he masturbates. Nor do the teens and preteens seduced by the fantasy that changing sex is possible have much in common with either of the other two groups.

Activists will tell you that people who call themselves trans were "born this way." But what way is that, exactly? How can transgenderism be a thing when it's so many disparate things? And how can "trans" people be "born this way" when most of those identifying as the opposite sex didn't imagine themselves having cross-sex alter egos until long after they were born? Even among those who are young enough to theoretically support the "born this way" claim, almost all will eventually embrace their natural sex, provided they aren't "transitioned" before that.

Transgenderism is internally and externally incoherent, inconsistent, and illogical.

But as long as those who make society's rules treat make-believe as if it were real, it will continue to have real consequences.

New government regulations and laws are wiping out speech, privacy, safety, and other rights related to sex. The dismantling of barriers between the sexes (and, indeed, between older men claiming trans identities and young girls) is an open invitation to opportunists, cheats, and sexual predators.

Just say you're trans and any door that was closed to you on account of sex opens wide.

Because trans ideology has so successfully infiltrated our society, it's also changed the rules we once lived by. And countless people are being tossed aside as collateral damage. In the next couple of chapters, you'll meet some of them.

Chapter 8

Males in Girls' Sports—
How Is This Fair?

"When you're not able to say out loud and in public that there are differences between men and women, the world has gone mad."

—Bari Weiss

Will could have been the poster boy for what social justice warriors decry as white male privilege. He was six feet, four inches of square-shouldered Texan, and he had it all: a well-to-do suburban upbringing, swimming lessons since the age of five, and after high school, entry into the rarefied world of the Ivy League. If Will didn't instantly attract the full measure of scorn from social justice warriors, it might have been because he wasn't, at first, prominent enough in his sport to get anyone's attention.

During the 2018–2019 school year, Will ranked 65th among all male college swimmers nationwide in the 500-yard freestyle, and just 554th in the 200-yard freestyle. He was never going to qualify for the Olympic trials. The NCAA championship, even more competitive, was out of reach.

So, what made the social justice crowd focus so sharply on this tall Texan, and more than that, see this pillar of privilege through an uber-approving lens during the Ivy Leaguer's final year? Why would they care that an also-swam, after a year's lay-off while Covid shut down everything, including college sports, was suddenly looking very much like a champion?

It was St. Patrick's Day, March 17, 2022, and ESPN was covering the NCAA Finals 500-freestyle. It began as a nail-biter. Then the announcer noted the Ivy Leaguer "pulling away over the final 150 meters . . . had to work for it . . . pushed the first 350 meters . . . " And then—a win! with the respectable, though far from record-breaking, time of 4:33.24.

Competing against the best of the best swimmers, the athlete with the Adonis-like body had shot from sixty-fifth place to first. It was an unusual victory that topped the times of three Olympians in the race who had, just six months before, taken home medals from Tokyo.

Depending on how you view this feat, you might call it a St. Patrick's Day miracle. Or you might assume that a long, Covid-imposed rest changed the odds. Or you might suspect something fishy.

Earlier that same season, Kim Jones, a former tennis pro and the mother of another Ivy League swimmer, had been surprised as she perused the preliminary swim meet results and saw a name she didn't recognize. This new-to-her swimmer was doing phenomenally well in the early meets.

Girls who were going to qualify for the NCAA championship meets later in the year typically swam around a 1:48 to 1:50 in practice meets for the 200-yard freestyle. This new young athlete had clocked a 1:46.

Great swimmers didn't just come out of nowhere. Who was this kid?

She checked the swim sites that show individual swimmer progress. She found this "new" swimmer had been competing throughout high school and for three years at the University of Pennsylvania.

On the male team.

Different name. Same individual.

In 2019, the swimmer was listed as Will Thomas. Now, after more than a year of cross-sex hormone therapy, he had changed names from Will to "Lia" and claimed a transgender identity.

Whatever was in Lia's mind, that mind was still housed in Will

Thomas's head and attached to Will Thomas's body. Lia had the same wide shoulder span. Lia had the same six-foot-four-inch frame. Lia still had a penis. Female hormones might have driven down Lia's testosterone levels, but hormones aren't the sum of what makes a body male or female. The athlete towered over his female competitors; two might fit in Lia's shadow.

What possessed Lia to leave the male team to join the girls? If we take Lia's word about the change in identity, again, the identity was in Lia's head. That identity never submerged itself in a pool with a bunch of young females. Lia's male body did that.

Lia's far more robust cardiovascular system pumped blood and oxygen to fuel that body in a way no girl's body could match. VO_2 max is the maximum rate of oxygen a body is able to use during exercise. (V is volume; O_2 is oxygen; max is maximum.) "Even truly elite women have VO_2 max values ~10% lower than those seen in men of similar elite status," note the authors of a study that demonstrated this deficit. And that's just the heart and lungs.

A 2021 study by researchers in Bologna, Italy, compared the bodies of male and female athletes on a number of other physical factors that affect athletic performance. All the athletes in the study had competed in strength and power events at the regional level in the year previous. Measuring the athletes' muscles using ultrasound, the researchers found that muscle thickness was significantly lower in the women: about 27 percent to about 45 percent lower than the males, depending on the site. In squats and weight-lifting tests, women's maximum strength was 53 to 59 percent lower than that of the male athletes.

Male and female bodies are different, and a prescription for cross-sex hormones can't undo that difference in any significant way.

Consider, for example, size.

Lia's long arms gave the athlete a male's wingspan in the water. Lia's hands operated as massive paddles to push the water behind the muscular male body slicing through it. Lia's male torso, after a lifetime of athletics, was so well-muscled, it resembled that of a Marvel superhero.

Lia knew all this about his body. Knew how it could perform, hormones notwithstanding. Knew the times and rankings of the other swimmers. Lia didn't need to read scientific research to understand the differences between male and female bodies' times in the pool, or that a mediocre time for a male swimmer could win a championship for a female one.

Lia Thomas also knew his own times had diminished only marginally after starting on estrogen.

As for the degree to which those cross-sex hormones affected Lia's performance, Kim has questions.

"Lia took time off of swimming during Covid," says Kim. "Most swimmers were committed to doing all they could to find water to swim in, and not give up any training ground."

If Lia took time off to focus on transitioning, that means that when the athlete complained about losing muscle mass since transitioning, it might have been partly or even mostly due to a lack of athletic training. Lia's times did drop somewhat in that period, but not enough to matter. As for his complaint about lost muscle mass? Well, just look at the guy.

When Lia was Will, he clocked his best 100-yard freestyle against other males at 47.15—too low to earn any rank at all, because it was outside that of the top 3,000 male swimmers. When later, as Lia, the swimmer competed in that same 100-yard freestyle against females with a time of 47.37, it was enough to rank among the top eight in the country.

The Ivy Leaguer's best 200-yard freestyle performance when swimming against males: 1:39.31. That gave Will a rank of 554. In the same competition against girls, the athlete's best time, 1:41.93, earned Lia fifth place, though it was less than 3 percent slower than Lia's best as a male (typical swim time differences between the sexes are 10 to 13 percent).

The swimmer's winning time in the 500-yard freestyle that saw Lia jet from sixty-fifth place to first was only about 6 percent slower than when competing as a male.

Trans activists have a phrase they use when asked how to handle touchy situations involving people who identify as trans: be kind.

But does being kind work both ways? Lia wasn't kind to the other swimmers and didn't care how his body's innate physical advantages would affect them. Lia only wanted to win.

The trans cult told Lia that this was fair. Having shed an oppressor identity, with it went all the rules that had previously applied. In the process, Lia Thomas had become heroic and viewed it as legitimate to express annoyance at anyone who might question what he was doing.

"They're using the guise of feminism to sort of push transphobic beliefs," Lia complained on the podcast of another swimmer who identified as trans. "I think a lot of people in that camp sort of carry an implicit bias against trans people."

In the current climate, it is possible to simultaneously take unfair advantage, to be applauded for doing so, and still be aggrieved.

Lia Thomas had taken undeserved places on the winners' podium, while managing to claim he was a victim.

Whatever you or I might think of Lia's choices, though, they're the choices of a college student, a kid who, despite his size, had not yet lived an independent adult life. Attending the University of Pennsylvania, a school saturated in queer theory concepts, the athlete was celebrated for every unsportsmanlike decision. Those decisions might have been different without that celebration and support.

It wasn't just UPenn. Lia was enabled by an academic system so ideologically captured that the coaches, athletic directors, national governing bodies, and other decision-makers seemed never to consider that hundreds of female swimmers also had rights. Those young athletes also had needs and hopes and expectations, all of which were being trampled by adults they trusted.

Aghast when she first realized Lia would be swimming against the college girls, Kim called her daughter Talia* and told her what she'd discovered. It was the first Talia had heard any of this. "That's not fair," she said, disappointment evident in her voice. But she was sure that the decision wouldn't stand. Those in charge, Talia believed, would figure out that they'd made a mistake, and all would be well. Kim was less optimistic.

"I spoke to almost every parent I came across. Everyone was upset and recognized the insanity of the situation. No one was okay with it—teammates' parents, club parents, parents in other sports, athletes in other sports, onlookers."

No one was okay with it, except those with decision-making authority. The only problem, in the view of the schools, was that the female collegiate swimmers and their families might publicly complain about their new teammate.

So the powers-that-be sent out a message to all the female swimmers that boiled down to this: head down; mouth zipped.

The Ivy League schools went further, condemning what they labeled "transphobia" and "hate" and announcing that they supported Lia Thomas.

Lia, meanwhile, was posting the fastest times in the country, in the female category, against actual females in mid-season travel meets, as all the swimming families were talking, worrying, and wondering what, if anything, they could do. Their daughters had trained almost their entire lives for these competitions.

The Ivy League schools called their female swimmers in for meetings and read off speeches that were similar in form and content.

After that, Talia called her mom in a panic. They all had to keep quiet, Talia said. If any harm came to any trans person, the schools had warned the girls, it would be their fault.

"This message of, 'You're going to be responsible for the suicide of another individual,' was coming down from people that they respected and trusted," said Kim, emotion rising in her voice. "These were their elders, their coaches, their leaders. These were people that they chose to follow by choosing to go to those schools. I couldn't believe that an adult could read that kind of language and not recognize that this was emotional blackmail and abuse. It was shocking to me."

Kim knew someone at the ACLU who handled litigation for Title IX cases. Title IX is the civil rights law that prohibits discrimination against girls in in any school, kindergarten through college, that receives federal funding. Its exact wording is: "No person in the United States shall, on the basis of sex, be excluded from participation in, be denied the benefits of, or be subjected to discrimination under any education program or activity receiving Federal financial assistance." It seems hard to believe today, but prior to Title IX's passage, some schools prohibited girls from taking courses that were considered male-oriented like calculus or shop. But what Title IX is best known for is opening up sports opportunities for girls that hadn't previously existed. Prior to its passage in 1972, about one in twenty-seven girls played sports. Now, about one in five do.

The activists' demand, "Let them play," make it seem as if males athletes who self-identify as female would be denied that right unless they are allowed to compete against the opposite sex. But that isn't true.

One of Talia's lifelong friends, a girl who'd begun identifying as a trans boy, was already on the female swimming team. Because Talia's friend was born female and had a female body, swimming with the rest of the girls had never caused any concerns about fairness. Whatever identity was in her head, the swimmer had none of the physical advantages of Lia Thomas.

The ACLU had been aggressively pushing the case for expanding the rights of those who called themselves transgender, but Kim was pretty sure that in this case, the female swimmers would find a champion at the organization. "I thought they were adamant defenders of women and women's rights."

She called her ACLU acquaintance, careful to refer to Lia by preferred pronouns but making her case that girls already have so many fewer opportunities in sports than boys. Allowing biological males to join their teams meant girls would lose even more of the precious few chances to compete that were guaranteed to them by Title IX. They'd lose their places on teams to those born male. They'd lose their scholarships. They deserved the right to keep their ranks limited just to biological females.

"I didn't for once think that [the ACLU] wouldn't recognize a conflict," says Kim. "It's so painfully obvious."

The lawyer shut Kim down almost immediately. It was wrong to use the words "genetic" and "biological," she said. Those words had no place in the vocabulary when referring to sex or gender.

"Transwomen are women," she told Kim. "They are female." The ACLU was, in fact, in the process of trying to remove any distinction in the legal language between sex and gender.

And that meant that no language that made any distinction between those born female and those males who imagined themselves to be a new gender would be tolerated by the organization.

But then, the lawyer said something that made it clear that that wasn't precisely the organization's position. Kim recalls her saying: "Let me tell you with certainty: the ACLU will never represent cis-women against women."

Stop there for a moment and process that comment. Kim is sure these were the lawyer's exact words because she wrote them down as they were spoken.

Humans who were born female didn't qualify as plain, ordinary "women" according to the lawyer's comment. Instead, they were "cis-women." Labeling them required a prefix to indicate which subcategory of women they belonged to.

Biological males who self-identified out of their sex, however, required no prefix to indicate their own subcategory because, according to the ACLU, unlike their cis-sisters, there was nothing "sub" about them. They were the main category. The males were no longer transwomen. They were simply "women."

"I think that conversation was like a baptism," says Kim, "an understanding of how important language is. Because it was that forty-five-minute conversation where I realized I have no language left to discuss this if I follow those rules."

Marshi Smith had been a collegiate swimmer at the University of Arizona, graduating in 2006. She'd won an NCAA championship title in the 100 backstroke, and earned All-American honors in numerous events. But by 2022, she had turned her attention to being a full-time mom.

"I was actually potty-training my three-year-old when collegiate swimming began unraveling with Lia Thomas's participation in women's swimming," she recalls. "And everything that I believed about justice and fairness and opportunities hit me in that blast-shattering moment."

She thought of her then six-year-old daughter who had started swim lessons that year. What would this mean for *her* future?

Marshi wrote letters to the University of Arizona athletic director and the president of the NCAA. With her history as a champion, she assumed that her words would carry weight. But two weeks later, as she watched Lia Thomas win the 500-free in the female category, Marshi still had gotten no response.

All Marshi's former teammates began group-texting, emailing, calling, messaging each other, alarmed at what was happening to the sport they loved, and trying to figure out what to do. One of Marshi's friends asked her to pen a group letter that they would all sign, thinking it might get more attention than individual ones.

They had to listen, right? Those who were making these decisions obviously didn't understand the sport. They hadn't considered any potential solutions other than putting a male body in the pool to compete against all the females.

With high hopes, women swim team members from the 1990s to the present, including forty heavy hitters—Olympic gold medalists, world champions, NCAA women of the year, and an NCAA coach of the year—sent their joint missive.

The response was . . . nothing. No response at all.

"Even our university athletic director refused to have a conversation with us," Marshi said. "I think the hopes of the NCAA and our university were just for it to quietly go away. But we were adamant about actually enacting change. None of us really understood. How did we get here?"

Marshi spent days on the phone trying to figure out who was ready to join this fight in earnest, and what they needed to do next.

She connected with Riley Gaines, a twelve-time All-American from the University of Kentucky, and one of the swimmers who Lia Thomas had competed against in the NCAA championships. Riley had tied Lia Thomas for fifth place in the 200-yard freestyle. But an NCAA official told Riley that there would be no trophy for her that day. There was only one available, and it would go to the male swimmer. Riley's, he said, would have to wait. They'd mail it. (A month later, it still hadn't arrived.)

It was perhaps the most disorienting moment in an already shocking season: a young athlete who'd earned her award through skill and sheer determination was told to step aside so a male almost twice her size could take the female competition prize.

It turned Riley Gaines into an activist.

Although Talia had begged Kim not to go public because of the veiled—and not-so-veiled—threats the girls had gotten about repercussions, Kim felt she could not keep silent. But she agreed that when she spoke out, she would do so anonymously. The first time she did so publicly was on February 26, 2022, at a Women's Declaration International webinar, identified only as "Mother of Swimmer, USA."

Soon after, Riley Gaines connected Kim with Marshi Smith.

Most stories in the media suggested that female college swimmers, other than a few malcontents, were happy with Lia Thomas on the female swim team. They realized that if they wanted to change the narrative, they needed a much bigger audience.

The National Association of Collegiate Directors of Athletics was holding a conference in Las Vegas on May 4, 2022. That's when they would make their push.

"We flew people in from South Africa, from England," says Kim, "and we had twelve Olympic gold medals in the front row alone in the audience."

Tennis great Martina Navratilova attended via Zoom as did track and field legend and Olympic Gold medalist Benita Mosley.

Meanwhile, although still feeling intimidated by those who controlled the world of college swimming, Talia agreed that her mother could go public under her own name. Their organization, formed to ensure that biological females got a seat at the table where the fate of female sports was being decided (because at that moment, only trans activists' voices were being heard), got its own name: The Independent Council On Women's Sports (ICONS).

"Everything just fell into place; it was perfect synergy," says Kim.

But it wasn't enough to simply advocate for girls and women in sports. Marshi and Kim realized that to find the way back, they had to retrace the steps that had taken female sports so far from its original purpose. After her conversation with the ACLU representative, Kim zeroed in on language. The trans movement began its push with what sounded like an innocuous premise: gender was separate from sex, a social construct that was distinct from the biological divide; "trans" people only wanted to be accepted as another gender, not another sex.

Treating gender as separate seemed like no big deal, and the least that empathic people could do.

Then, the movement began to conflate sex and gender, using the words interchangeably. And in the ACLU call, Kim learned the new goal—erase the line between male and female altogether.

To defend the rights of women and girls, they, too, had to focus on words. Because words weren't all that were being redefined.

ICONS speaks for female athletes who aren't always able to speak up for themselves because of the risk to sponsorships, placements on teams, and "cancellation" beyond their athletic careers.

It's not easy getting their message to people who have been sold a false narrative by media that's been mostly captured by the trans movement, but they are making progress. A June 2023 Gallup poll found that the majority of Americans were against males competing in female sports. A January 2025 *New York Times* poll found much the same.

But you wouldn't suspect that if you listened to and read mainstream media sources.

In one NPR interview, for example, an expert claimed that it's merely a matter of prejudice to "target 'women' who have either a different biology or . . . simply look different."

That's a direct quote. The expert acknowledged that "men have, on average, an advantage in performance in athletics of about ten to twelve percent over women," but immediately questioned whether that gave male bodies an *actual* advantage in competition.

Spoiler alert: yes, it does, and that advantage is, minimum, about what he quoted—though some studies have found the average difference to be far greater. In certain sports, the advantages males have over females is profound. For example, according to a 2021 study published in the journal *Sports Medicine,* "The power produced during a punch was 162% greater in males than in females, and the least powerful man produced more power than the most powerful woman." (Despite this, two boxers who were proven to be male by DNA tests showing they each had XY chromosomes were allowed to fight females in the 2024 Olympics. Both males took home Olympic gold medals meant for women after pummeling female competitors.)

An analysis done by two faculty members of Duke University Law School, Doriane Coleman and Wickliffe Shreve, quantified how profound the differences in sports performance between the sexes can be. They found that in just one year, 2017: "Olympic, World, and U.S. Champion Tori Bowie's 100 meters lifetime best of 10.78 was beaten 15,000 times by men and boys."

It was much the same when they looked at another female Olympic champion's personal best performance in the 400-meter of 49.26. "Just in the single year 2017, men and boys around the world outperformed [Allyson Felix] more than 15,000 times."

These women were Olympic bronze, silver, and gold medalists. And yet, if their competitions had been open to both males and females, many thousands of males would have bested them. These champions never would have made it onto the field.

If major media outlets ignore how girls are being pushed out of their own teams and being denied the honors they rightfully won, ICONS has been keeping track.

"There is such a clear scientific and logical understanding that male performance in athletics is different than female performance," says Marshi, "which is why if you can convince society that in a place where we have kids—again, kids have an understanding of fairness between men and women's sports—if you can convince society that actually, no, men's bodies are the same as women's even in this category, then you can convince them of every other part of the ideology: in prisons, rape crisis centers, in bathroom facilities. Sport is so visible, it's so tangible to parents watching our kids perform and our own experiences as athletes. If you can infiltrate sports, you can infiltrate any part of society with this concept that men can be women and should have access to everything that a woman has."

As if to punctuate her comments, on July 14, 2022, the University of Pennsylvania nominated Lia Thomas for the NCAA Woman of the Year Award.

Girls who want to play sports are perhaps the largest group to be trampled as collateral damage as the trans craze sweeps through schools. Boys are competing against girls in middle school and high school sports in almost all categories.

But maybe, it's wrong to think of them as collateral damage, says psychotherapist Grace Ellison. Maybe, for some boys, getting the chance to beat—and in the sports that involve physical contact, beat up—girls is the point. In what other situation would a boy with anger against girls be applauded for hurting them?

In a Massachusetts girls' high school basketball game in April 2024, a six-foot-tall bearded boy who claimed to identify as a transgender girl injured three different girls during the first half of the game. Their coach decided to forfeit the game prior to playing the second half. It was simply too dangerous to continue.

Something similar happened in a girls' high school rugby match in Guam. One boy, claiming to be trans, injured three girls from the opposing team during the season's opening game. "The aggressive nature that was witnessed clearly showed that it's a definite issue that we have to deal with," the coach from the team with the injured girls was quoted as saying.

In other sports, though there might not be a direct risk of injury from aggression, there are other concerns.

In Connecticut, between 2017 and 2019, two boys who self-identified as trans were awarded fifteen women's state track championship titles. Along with losing races to the males, the girls on the high school track and field team lost the college scholarship opportunities that typically go to winning athletes. For some, that could mean losing the chance to go to college at all.

In May 2024, a male teenager won the 200-meter female Track and Field State Championships in Oregon. He got booed by the crowd. Less than two weeks later, in neighboring Washington state, a male took the top prize in the 400-meter female Track and Field State Championships. The girls cheered and clapped as the second-place finisher, a girl, took her place on the podium. When the boy who'd stolen first took his place, the girls silently put their hands behind their backs, and boos could be heard from the bleachers.

This overt disapproval marks a change, but it hasn't slowed the entry of males into girls' sports. So many males are taking championships from females, it's become impossible to keep track.

And there's more to consider when boys muscle their way into girls' sports than the game itself.

In a small town in Vermont, Blake Allen, a fourteen-year-old girl who played on the middle school volleyball team, walked into the girls' locker room, saw a boy, and walked right out. The boy was a fourteen-year-old who identified as trans—and who apparently had dressed and undressed with the girls' team. Blake told the school she was uncomfortable with this development and when doing so, used the word "boy."

First, the school staff told Blake there was nothing they could do and later, when she persisted in repeating her complaints, she was suspended from school for "misgendering." The school also ordered her to do a restorative justice circle—an event where a person who emotionally injures another works to heal the harm and restore harmony—and to write a letter of apology. Blake refused. She told them to go ahead and suspend her, but she wouldn't agree to the other terms. She'd done nothing wrong.

Her father, Travis Allen, was the school's soccer coach. When he learned what had happened to his daughter, he confronted the mother of the boy on social media, writing, in part: "The truth is your son watched my daughter and multiple other girls change in the locker room. While he got a free show, they got violated."

For that post, the school accused him, too, of misgendering and suspended Travis without pay.

But, unlike in most other instances where males join female sports teams and share facilities without any pushback, Travis Allen decided to sue.

The school has since dropped their suspensions and paid the family a settlement of $125,000.

Travis made the assumption that a male, however that person identified, would experience the same sexual arousal when watching girls undressing as most other males. Perhaps the school made the opposite assumption: that the trans student, identifying as a girl, would be only attracted to boys. Most people tend to assume that men who self-identified as transwomen would be gay guys if they didn't identify out of their sex.

Vermont law requires that schools allow kids to use facilities aligned with their gender identities. It's a good bet that legislators wrote that law after hearing from activists, but without considering how it might affect other students, and without realizing that despite the almost universal linking of LGB and T, sexual identity is separate from sexuality. One doesn't necessarily tell you about the other.

As noted in the previous chapter, autogynephilia and transvestic fetishism are sexual disorders. Those with autogynephilia are heterosexual males who fetishize the idea of themselves as women. For a small fraction, their sole object of attraction is themselves, but the vast majority are also attracted to women and girls. In earlier times people who had such kinks kept them in the closet to avoid stigma. But the current trans craze has coaxed such men into florid public display.

So, what does this have to do with intact biological males sharing locker rooms with female athletes?

Recall that Ray Blanchard and Michael Bailey, two experts who have studied those who identify as transgender, estimated that about 75 percent of males who currently identify as the opposite sex are heterosexual.

That's an awful lot of kinksters, almost all of whom still have their penises, most of whom have other fetishes, and the vast majority of whom are sexually attracted to girls and women. Does it make sense to coerce females into undressing in front of them? We're not talking about boys here, but full-grown men who game the system to gain access to girls.

In December 2023, a Canadian news outlet, *Rebel News*, was alerted to an oddly disturbing situation. At a swim meet for teen girls, one of the competitors was fifty years old. This swimmer, Nick, wore a woman's bathing suit that covered everything from chest to thighs, but under that clinging attire, onlookers could see outlines of an anatomy that was at odds with the swimmer's declared gender identity.

Why weren't any adults stepping in to protest?

Maybe it's because in an age partly governed by rules laid down by mass psychogenic madness, nobody knows what the rules are any more. Those who dare to challenge even wildly inappropriate behavior could easily find themselves punished for objecting. And, indeed, the community center's officials threatened to call police to eject *Rebel News* for filming, even though a number of others recording video of the swim meet on their phones at the same time were left undisturbed. It's also likely that the fear of being shamed for "transphobia" overcame, not just common sense, but other adults' instincts to protect young girls from an older man who might have had predatory inclinations.

Rebel News reported that Nick identified as a teen girl. But that doesn't appear to be accurate. Nick merely competes against teen girls—and has since at least 2019. In an October 2023 race, for example, Nick swam in a teen competition against eight girls; five were thirteen years old and the other three were fourteen. Nick's biography on the website of the college where he teaches notes that Nick and his wife have a "lesbian" relationship—a sign that Nick is autogynephilic.

It also seems that Nick was doing more than competing. The community center where the swim meet was held has both gender neutral and sex-segregated facilities available. Nick bypassed the gender-neutral and men's rooms, choosing, instead, to strip naked and change into street clothes in the same changing room where the young girls undressed.

"If a person truly has gender dysmorphic disorder, the last thing they want is for someone to see their genitalia," says psychotherapist Grace Ellison*. "So, if a man says he is a woman and therefore has the right to be in spaces just for women, and then exposes his intact male genitals while in that space, he is not suffering from an identity issue. He has an agenda."

Privacy, common sense, safeguarding—all are being abandoned because males who self-identify as the opposite sex compete with females and share their private spaces, including guys who have no illusions that they're anything but guys. Not all males are skilled enough to compete with other males. But against females?

How tempting might that look to a mediocre male athlete?

"Mom, there's this trans person on our team," Alicia* told Bridget* after returning from the first day of the 2021 rowing season. "And we all think he's a fake."

Kendall*, the so-called trans person, was over six feet tall, had a full, bushy beard, donned a male's swimming uniform for rowing practice, and changed into boy's clothes after. Alicia knew other kids who identified as trans; almost everyone did in their ultra-liberal area. But those males dressed in feminine styles. They shaved their faces, their legs, their arms, and their armpits. Kendall seemed quite content to be hairy all over.

Because Kendall went to a different school, Alicia didn't know whether her new teammate identified as trans outside of crew. But it wouldn't have mattered. There were no rules requiring a male to live as a female, or to identify as one anywhere else.

Could it be possible that Kendall didn't actually identify as the opposite sex?

"You're not allowed to ask," says Bridget.

It would require either mind-reading, or Kendall making an overt statement, one way or the other.

Bridget and another of the rowing moms decided they had to get some answers from the boathouse administration. Their concerns were essentially blown off.

Bridget had been thrilled when Alicia first started rowing in ninth grade at the age of fourteen. She'd been a timid child and had been bullied at school, never quite fitting in with the in-crowd. Crew changed all that for her. The rowing team practiced together six days a week and because they relied upon each other so completely in the boat, their bonds of friendship became strong. The camaraderie was unlike anything Alicia had previously experienced. She'd bloomed into a confident young woman, looking forward to the day she'd be chosen for the "1V" boat—the lead varsity boat—which would increase her chances for a scholarship.

"Rowing was the lodestone around which Alicia's life revolved," says Bridget. "She was very, very good at school but she loved crew even more."

Kendall had performed poorly the previous season on the boys' team and didn't seem interested in competing any more diligently this season. So, despite the boy's muscle mass that allowed him to row faster than anyone else, the coach decided against placing him in the 1V boat. That meant that the girls' biggest concerns about competition weren't realized.

But there was still the matter of the locker room. The administration wouldn't budge: Kendall had as much right to use it as any other member of the team.

In effect, that made Kendall the only one using it. Rather than disrobe in front of their bearded teammate, all the girls changed in their cars.

Nor did the administration see any issue with maintaining the usual protocol for away competitions: four girls to a hotel room; two girls to a bed.

Bridget says the coach, who was sympathetic to the plight of the majority on his team, struck a deal with the mom of one girl whose family was a bit more "bohemian" than others: Kendall and she would share a hotel room, and each would get a separate bed.

But the issue of Kendall's true identity came up again when the team was away for the second regatta of the spring season.

In each boat, there is a place for a coxswain who sits at the front and steers. Typically, this role goes to one of the smallest members of the team; it's often a girl even on the boys' team.

"Fraternization is an absolute no-no," says Bridget. "It is part of the athlete code of conduct that they sign every year. The parents also sign it. There is no fraternization within the team, outside the team, between the other teams."

Disobey this rule, the girls are told, and you're off the team. Immediately.

Yet, when Alicia came home from that regatta, she told her parents that Kendall had been making out with the female coxswain of one of the boys' teams. There were photos, taken by the coxswain's roommate.

Word got back to the coach, but the photos, apparently, did not. When he confronted Kendall, the presumed trans-rower said it had never happened. Alicia and all the other girls on the team who had seen the pictures were outraged. Why did the rules apply to all of them but not to this one team member? Was this the way the administration interpreted equality?

About a week later, one of Alicia's closest friends fell in the river during practice, got soaked, and had to go to the locker room for towels. Another of the girls accompanied her inside.

She was removing her sports bra when Kendall appeared, gaped at her, and exclaimed, "Ooooh, titties!"

Mortified, the half-naked girl quickly threw something over herself and rushed out sobbing, feeling dirty and insisting that it was all her own fault. She said she should have known better than to change in the locker room. That space, due to the trans-preference rules, had been exclusively Kendall's domain.

Wanting to forget it ever happened, the girl refused to tell any of the adults. But when the friend who'd been with her told their teammates, the others weren't so reticent. Alicia informed Bridget. Bridget told another of the moms. And, together, they confronted the boathouse's athletic director.

The athletic director already had learned of the incident and had contacted SafeSport, an organization that oversees safety for athletes who are minors. Within two days, Kendall was suspended for a year.

Kendall was gone but nothing had really changed. The next "Kendall" would be welcome and would encounter no more restrictions than the first. Perhaps by now, the same bearded Kendall is back and dominating the girls' sport.

Girls cannot count on having privacy or safety any longer. And, of course, as Marshi Smith noted, the intrusion is not confined to athletic spaces.

More about that in the next chapter.

Chapter 9

Why Are We Letting Males Invade Female-Only Spaces?

US Senator Marsha Blackburn:
"Can you provide a definition for the word 'woman'?"

Judge Ketanji Brown Jackson:
"Can I provide a definition? No. I can't. Not in this context.
I'm not a biologist."

—Senate Supreme Court Confirmation Hearing

At noon on May 28, 2021, a fifteen-year-old girl visited the girl's bathroom at Stone Bridge High School in Loudoun County, Virginia. She was there to meet another ninth-grader: a boy who was dressed in girl's clothing. The two had had consensual sex two weeks previously.

They were together in the handicapped toilet stall when a teacher's assistant entered the bathroom and noticed two sets of feet under the stall's door. The teacher's assistant said nothing and did nothing; she would later say that she assumed there was an innocent reason for what she saw. Here is what a Special Grand Jury reported about that day and its aftermath:

- The boy had become aggressive toward the girl. He held down her arms and penetrated her anally.
- When the teacher's assistant walked in, the boy jumped up.
- The girl, now in pain, rose more slowly.
- The boy pushed down her shoulders and grabbed her face.
- Once the teacher's assistant had left, he forced the girl to perform fellatio on him.
- The boy disappeared somewhere in the school while the girl went to school officials to tell them that she'd been raped.
- The school called her parents, Scott and Jessica Smith, telling them only that their daughter had been assaulted.
- Scott arrived at the school at 2:15 p.m., but the "school resource officer" (a euphemism for a law enforcement officer whose beat is inside a public school) would not allow Smith to enter because the father didn't bring identification with him.
- Scott phoned Jessica, who was already with their child, and Jessica told him it wasn't just an assault. Their daughter had been raped.
- Horrified and enraged, Scott, still trying to get to his child and being thwarted by the officer, caused "a scene."
- The officer finally escorted Scott inside at 2:30 p.m.

Almost anyone would understand that a parent, learning of an attack on his teen daughter, would be upset, even enraged—doubly so, when he was prevented from rushing to her side. By itself, this incident would be traumatic. But the school system made it more so.

According to the grand jury report, the officials involved appeared to have done everything in their power to cover up the rape. It also appears that they did so for one key reason: they believed the rapist was trans.

Later that afternoon, Kevin Lewis, the chief operating officer of Loudoun County Public Schools, arrived at Stone Bridge High School. After conferring with Principal Timothy Flynn, Lewis sent out a video-conferencing meeting announcement to senior staff. All the information it gave, other than this was to be an update, and the scheduled time, was that the subject to be addressed was that, "The incident at SBHS is related to policy 8040."

Policy 8040 concerned the rights of transgender and gender-expansive students. It was not yet the district's official policy, and a large contingent of parents opposed it. A school board meeting to hear testimony from parents and other interested parties about the proposed policy was to be held in about three weeks, on June 22, 2021.

How would it look if, right at the moment when school officials were pushing to allow trans kids to use the bathrooms that matched their "gender identities," word got out that a "gender fluid" boy raped a girl in one of those same girls' bathrooms? It certainly wouldn't help them to pass Policy 8040, especially since the boy was wearing a skirt when he did it.

The administrators could read between the lines of that brief cryptic email from Lewis and recognize what was at stake.

Much later, when speaking to the grand jury, Principal Flynn, who'd joined Lewis's videoconference late, recalled that the others wanted to hear from him directly about what had happened. Not one of the other attendees claimed to recall what topic was discussed during that meeting. The grand jury report labeled this "intentional amnesia."

One of those administrators, school superintendent Scott Ziegler, emailed members of the school board that there had been an alleged sexual assault at the school. He conveniently left out any mention of Policy 8040. He also conveniently neglected to say that the boy was dressed as a girl.

A different email, composed by the school system's public relations department and edited by Ziegler, was sent to parents. Although Principal Flynn didn't write it, the email was sent with his signature from his account. This email went much further in covering up what had happened. It was clearly intended to convince parents that anything they might have heard about an incident at the school involved just a minor kerfuffle.

The email made no mention of a sexual assault.

It claimed that "there was no threat to the safety of the student body."

The email acknowledged that the county sheriff had dispatched deputies to the school but suggested that that was because of the angry exchange that some students overheard between Scott Smith and the school's resource officer.

Otherwise, nothing to see here, folks.

It's clear from yet another email, this one actually written by Flynn, that the sexual assault wasn't their primary concern. In it, he noted that

Scott Smith had created "quite a show that scared and intimidated students and staff."

Flynn's email said they probably should have had Smith arrested.

There was no mention, in any of these communications, of having the rapist in the skirt arrested.

The Loudoun County Sheriff "did not see fit" to take the boy into custody, failed to collect much evidence, and without explanation, told others they considered it a shaky case. Unfortunately, it's not that unusual for cops to shrug off sexual assault allegations. It's also not unusual for law enforcement to let rape kits pile up in their evidence lockers, untested. It's not even unheard of for them to discard untested rape kits when police departments decide that they need to "make space" for evidence in other cases.

When classes resumed after the Memorial Day weekend, the school made just one adjustment. The rapist and his victim were kept separate from each other. That was it.

The grand jury report noted that the boy was back on his school computer that day, "deleting conversations—and potentially evidence—from Discord."

Fast forward to June 22, 2021, and the Loudoun County school board meeting to discuss, among other issues, the school district's proposed new policy of allowing biological male students to use the girls' bathrooms.

Scott and Jessica Smith were among those attending. Smith, a burly man, his fair hair mostly gone, had never been to one of these meetings before. But this one was important. The school system was covering up what happened to his child.

Other parents, who knew nothing of the sexual assault, came to oppose the transgender policy or the introduction of critical race theory into the school district's policies, or both. A number of them demanded that Ziegler stop fighting an order to reinstate a popular teacher, Tanner Cross, who the superintendent had fired for speaking out against Policy 8040 and Policy 8350, which would allow biological males who identified as girls to use the girls' locker rooms and participate in girls' sports.

Parents lined up around the block. Inside, it was a packed house. And raucous. Several held up red cardboard signs with white lettering that said "We the Parents Stand Up."

People cheered and booed. Some shouted demands for Ziegler's resignation.

Smith, though he didn't request one, was given a ticket so that he could join the queue of parents and others—259 in all—waiting to comment.

If you saw only the first twenty minutes of the comment period, you'd imagine that the majority of speakers supported Policy 8040. But after those first speakers, most who stepped up to the lectern did so to protest during their allotted one minute. A few complained about how poorly students were doing in school; although the district was adept at requiring lessons that were influenced by critical race theory and gender theory, it was failing at teaching kids to do math at grade level. Only 64 percent were proficient.

But many more were worried about the safety of girls when biological males had carte blanche to enter their previously private single-sex spaces.

A plump blonde school board member, her black V-neck sweater showing off the string of pearls around her neck, tried to assuage parents' concerns by asking Superintendent Ziegler whether there were, in fact, reports of bathroom or locker room assaults on a regular basis. She, like other school board members, would have known that there was at least one such report because she'd received Ziegler's email about the attack on the Smiths' daughter. Nevertheless, Ziegler didn't hesitate to tell a bald-faced lie: "We don't have any record of assaults occurring in our restrooms." Parents' responses indicated they were not, in fact, assuaged. Here's a representative sampling of public comments:

I'm [name], a mother of two daughters and two sons and a sexual assault survivor. I am here to plead with you to stop the push for 8040 and 8350 as they fail to protect all students.

Why is indoctrination allowed to take place under your watch? Why is continued misinformation allowed to be distributed under your watch? Why is only a one-way narrative allowed to take place under your watch?

I have three children in LCPS. My oldest child will be starting mid-

dle school in the fall. Where is her protection if a biological male is staring at her as she changes her clothes in the locker room? Where is her protection if she runs track and loses every time to a biological male? Where is the protection for teachers forced to call students a pronoun that does not match their biology?

We have separate bathrooms because of what our bodies do in them. Bodies matter. Calling girls bigots because they don't want to use the toilet in a stall next to a boy or get undressed next to a boy is cruel and wrong. It is embarrassing enough for a girl to change a pad knowing all the other girls can hear the crinkle of the packaging. But telling her that she must be okay doing it in the presence of boys because their preferred pronouns are "she/her"? How evil can you be?

I have taught precious teenagers who identify as transgender. I chose to address them respectfully by using their preferred first name, not their pronoun. It is possible to teach and be kind without affirming. No child should be taught to demand another's affirmation.

If I declare I'm a woman today, can I follow you into the woman's bathroom? This is a school building after all. Can you be followed into a locker room before gym and be watched as you change into gym clothes, since this is allowed in middle school?

I'm retired Senator Dick Black of Ashburn, Virginia . . . it's absurd and immoral for teachers to call boys girls and girls boys. You're making teachers lie to students. And even kids know that it's wrong. This board has a dark history of suppressing free speech. They caught you red-handed with an enemies' list to punish opponents of critical race theory. You're teaching children to hate others because of their skin color, and you're forcing them to lie about other kids' gender. I am disgusted by your bigotry . . .

Someone appears to have cut off the former state senator's mic at this point because he sounded like he was in mid-sentence when his audio went silent. Audience members shouted, waved their signs, and some gave the senator a standing ovation. A board member could be heard saying, "Madam Chair, I move to end public comment." And that's what the school board abruptly did to a resounding round of boos from the crowd.

Some in the audience left while many if not most milled around talking to one another. The Smiths told their story of rape and cover-up to others standing nearby.

An acquaintance of the Smiths, a woman with long dark hair, wearing a white T-shirt with a heart-shaped rainbow pattern in the middle, vehemently insisted to Jessica Smith that the bathroom attack on her daughter had never happened. Scott Smith, wearing an old gray T-shirt with the logo of his plumbing company, Plumb Crazy, on the back, stepped in and bluntly told her otherwise.

According to Scott Smith's later testimony, that's when the acquaintance threatened to ruin his business on social media.

Smith let loose with a stream of profanity. A deputy grabbed him from behind. Smith tried to pull away. Two deputies tackled him and wrestled him to the floor. Other deputies piled on, scattering the metal-framed red-cushioned chairs that had been set up for the meeting. Within moments, the bloodied and dazed father was dragged across the floor, handcuffed, and forcibly removed from the room as his wife cried out, "My child was raped at school and this is what happens?"

Shock rippled through the room as other parents learned about the sexual assault allegations. A few days after his arrest, Scott Smith went public with his accusations on social media.

The sheriff's department finally took the rapist into custody on July 10, 2021. The adolescent spent fourteen days at a juvenile detention center before being released with an ankle bracelet to await trial. His probation officer determined that the assailant could not go back to Stone Bridge High School. So, the school district, without apparent concern for possible consequences, transferred him to a different school, Broad Run High School, never notifying parents that this was the same "gender fluid" boy who'd allegedly raped a girl in a Stone Bridge High School bathroom. Only the principal at the new school knew that the boy was awaiting trial for sexual assault. And he showed a remarkable lack of curiosity about the details.

Meanwhile, on August 11, 2021, the school board, despite the public pleas of the majority of Loudoun County parents, voted to make Policy

8040 official.

After the school year began at Broad Run High School, a couple of girls complained about their new classmate's creepy stalking behavior toward them. But no one knew there was a reason to be on high alert.

On October 6, 2021, the boy struck again. He grabbed a girl in the hallway, pulled her into an empty classroom, and put her in a chokehold, nearly asphyxiating her so he could sexually assault her.

This time, there could be no coverup.

With the boy once again arrested, media quickly figured out this was the "gender fluid" rapist from Stone Bridge High. He was charged with abduction and sexual battery while still awaiting sentencing after having been found guilty in the bathroom rape for two counts of forcible sodomy, one count of anal sodomy, and one count of forcible fellatio. Remanded to a juvenile facility, the Loudoun County high school rapist was released from court supervision on his eighteenth birthday.

For his handling of the situation and the cover-up, Superintendent Scott Ziegler was fired.

But a zealous prosecutor was still going after Scott Smith for what happened at the school board meeting, apparently to make an example of him. Just days before the second sexual assault, the National School Boards Association, which represents school boards across the country, sent a letter to the White House suggesting that parents who disrupt school board meetings were dangerous and should be thought of as possible domestic terrorists. They asked that the FBI and Department of Homeland Security, among other agencies, investigate such parents.

The letter specifically pointed to Smith's arrest at the June 22, 2021, meeting, and linked to an article that claimed (erroneously, apparently, but the damage was done) that he had physically threatened someone.

Despite public revelations of what had occurred, several school officials were still doing their best to conceal many of the details surrounding the rape of the Smiths' daughter, claiming to the grand jury that the boy wasn't actually dressed as a girl but was wearing a kilt. The ploy didn't work. The report from the grand jury was scathing concerning officials' attempts to obfuscate and deceive.

In September 2023, Virginia Governor Glenn Youngkin finally pardoned Scott Smith.

Would school officials have handled this incident differently if the boy were wearing pants instead of a skirt? From the grand jury report, it seems likely that school officials attempted to hide the truth in order to reduce pushback against the passage of Policy 8040. Public disclosure of a rape by a "gender fluid" student probably would have made passage politically impossible.

But as long as no one knew, the narrative could be presented as feasible:

- Males invading the single-sex spaces of females couldn't possibly pose a threat to anyone because their anatomy is meaningless;
- All that counts is what they claim is in their heads;
- They're oppressed and their motives are pure;
- "Transgirls" are girls, and they just want to pee.

Any evidence to the contrary must be buried. Any accuser must be silenced.

A fourteen-year-old rapist in a skirt blew apart that carefully constructed narrative. He *was* a threat. And he sure didn't just want to pee.

In an interesting plot twist, the rapist's mother later reportedly claimed that her son had been faking his trans identity. She said that he only wore women's clothes, and claimed to be "gender fluid," to get attention. He was just a boy who wanted sex.

The problem isn't that all males are predatory. Far from it.

The problem is that predators exist. They don't wear signs around their necks to identify themselves. But they're always on the lookout for the means to land their prey.

They rely on camouflage, stalking prey from inside the herd, hoping you'll mistake them for another type of beast with similar spots and stripes.

Schools are giving predators easy access because of outlandish ideas about gender and sex that no one would have taken seriously even a decade ago. And it's not just schools.

What did he have to lose? That appears to be what James Tubbs asked himself in early 2022 when DNA matched him to a cold case: the 2014 sexual assault in a California Denny's restaurant bathroom of a ten-year-old girl. He'd sneaked into the women's room, grabbed the terrified child by the throat, and yanked her into a stall. There, he molested her, shoving his hand into her underwear and forcing her to do what he wanted. Had another customer not entered the women's room while he was sexually tormenting the child, there's little doubt that he would have done worse. Cameras captured his image as he fled, but at the time, he wasn't identified.

It hadn't been his first sexual attack on a child. The year prior, he'd exposed himself to a four-year-old in a California library while her mother was browsing titles just a couple of aisles away. He groped her, attempting to get her to touch his exposed genitals. He seemed to believe she'd be too afraid to escape while he raced to the customer service desk to retrieve the bathroom key. But as soon as he turned away, the tiny child ran screaming and crying to her mother, pointing to her mouth and genitals as she sobbed out the details of the attack.

Though police arrived and the four-year-old identified Tubbs, for some reason, he was never prosecuted.

In the intervening eight years, Tubbs accrued a long record of other crimes, some violent, and probation violations.

It was after his conviction in 2020 for a stabbing that his DNA finally got entered into the federal CODIS database. That tied him to the 2014 cold case involving the ten-year-old he'd molested.

Though Tubbs could talk his way out of a lot of things, his DNA spoke louder. That didn't mean he was without recourse. While in custody, awaiting trial, jailhouse recordings captured the voices of Tubbs and his father scheming to limit his time behind bars. They came up with a ploy tailored to the age of trans insanity.

Los Angeles District Attorney George Gascón, touting himself as a progressive, announced a range of reformist policies that he promised to implement from day one. Among those policies was his refusal to charge minors as adults. James Tubbs was currently twenty-six—long in the tooth for a juvenile justice proceeding. He had been just two weeks shy of eighteen years old when he attacked the ten-year-old. But maybe, the scales of justice could be tipped if they played the trans card. Edward Tubbs, James's father, communicated James's new name to his inmate son on the tapped jailhouse phone line—a name that James clearly had not chosen for himself, nor even heard before that moment:

> *Edward Tubbs:* Hey, uh, uh, Hannah.
> *James Tubbs:* Huh?
> *Edward Tubbs:* (firmly) Hannah.
> *James Tubbs:* (sounding confused) Yes?

The younger Tubbs was catching on but the elder Tubbs wanted to make sure. Edward explained that he'd gotten a call from his son's lawyer and the lawyer reported that she now was representing, not James, but "Hannah" Tubbs.

Edward jokingly told his incarcerated son that he would have preferred the lawyer renaming him Jamie. But the precise moniker really didn't matter. The "identity" was everything.

In his mug shot, James's beard and moustache left no doubt that he was a he. He had never before pretended to be anything other than male. Still, he had everything to gain and nothing to lose. So, why not? If lived experience was all that counted, James Tubbs now had about five minutes of lived experience as trans—more than enough—and a new name to make it official. He'd joined the oppressed. Anyone who said otherwise would be a bigot. Not even Fox News dared call James "him" when they reported on his case. The network dutifully labeled him a transgender woman named Hannah, complete with she/her pronouns.

DA Gascón knew of James Tubbs's vile past. His department also knew of the jailhouse recordings that showed this new trans identity was a sham. Nevertheless, Gascón offered a plea deal to the thug because, he claimed, that as a "transgender woman," Tubbs would be at risk of assault in an adult prison. If Tubbs pled guilty, Gascón would arrange for him to be prosecuted, not as an adult, but as a minor.

A *female* minor.

James Tubbs jumped at the deal.

Because it was a juvenile court matter, this serial child molester wouldn't be required to register as a sex offender upon release. He would serve just two years total, with the year he'd already spent in custody counted toward his sentence. He'd be housed in the juvenile justice system in a facility for girls, his preferred victims.

To the sane observer, the Gascón's decision looked (to use the technical term), batshit crazy.

That's how it appeared to Shea Sanna, the prosecutor assigned to the case. It seemed even more so, soon after, when Tubbs was charged with an additional crime, committed in 2019: bludgeoning a friend to death with a rock in a dispute over some money Tubbs stole. (His father was also charged for intimidating witnesses in the case.)

Sanna sounded the alarm, publicly revealing that he had recordings of the conspiracy to give Tubbs a new name and fake trans identity. You'd think that that would make the prosecutor a hero, right?

But in the upside-down world we now live in, what mattered most was not Tubbs's crimes, but prosecutor Sanna's own offense. Sanna, when publicly revealing the plot, had "dead-named" the prisoner and "misgendered" him. That was crime enough to get the prosecutor suspended from his job.

Operating under a provably wrong assumption that those who identify as trans must always be seen as the victims, never as victimizers, our society is knocking down all the barriers between predator and prey.

If we can't protect children, or punish those who sexually abuse them, imagine what dangers we're subjecting vulnerable adults to. Actually, there's no need to imagine. Here's a sampling of what's been happening, not just in the United States but in other places where the ideology has taken hold.

In 2015, the UK House of Commons presented the British Psychological Society with a wide-ranging inquiry about transgender equality. The legislators were concerned whether trans-identifying people were being treated fairly in the prison system. The psychological society responded, but added its own list of different concerns:

> [P]sychologists working with forensic patients are aware of a number of cases where **men convicted of sex crimes have falsely claimed to be transgender females** [emphasis added] for a number of reasons:

- *As a means of demonstrating reduced risk and so gaining parole;*
- *As a means of explaining their sex offending aside from sexual gratification (e.g., wanting to "examine" young females);*
- *Or as a means of separating their sex offending self (male) from their future self (female).*
- *In rare cases it has been thought that the person is seeking better access to females and young children through presenting in an apparently female way.*

It's not clear why the last reply was qualified with the term "in rare cases." It's possible that while inmates interviewed by prison psychologists admitted freely to the first several motivations, they were less willing to admit to the last and most obvious one. The society's response to British lawmakers went on to add that giving sex-offending inmates estrogen or blocking androgen wouldn't necessarily reduce the risk of them continuing to commit sex crimes. It urged the government not to change its policies in ways that would allow some of the most dangerous people in society "greater latitude to offend."

But, despite these warnings, parts of the United Kingdom did change prison policies to ensure "transgender equality." They began allowing males who claimed to be trans, no matter what the crime, to be housed with women on a "case-by-case basis." In Scotland, "case-by-case" seems to have translated roughly to: "Sure, why not?"

Scotland's population is just 5.5 million, about that of Minnesota. It incarcerates about 5,600 post-conviction prisoners. Of those, in 2023, nineteen men claimed to be trans.

Funny thing, though: only seven of those prisoners had called themselves trans prior to arrest and conviction. The other twelve—the majority—had never shown an interest in asserting a new gender identity until after they were caught committing whatever crimes they committed.

Few Scots seemed to be paying much attention to how all this might play out in the justice system until the case of "Isla Bryson" made headlines. "Isla" had been convicted in January 2023 of two rapes, one in 2016 and another in 2019, and was being held at Scotland's only women's prison while awaiting sentencing.

When going by the names Adam Graham and Adam Bryson, the stocky Scot—shaved head, tattooed face—had been arrested in 2019.

While out on bail, Adam began claiming to be transgender, using the name Isla Annie Bryson. He got himself a blonde wig that swept the side of his face, partly obscuring some of the tattoos, and enrolled in a beauty school course. There, he used the name "Annie." Among other lessons, he and his classmates took a spray tanning class. "Annie" seemed particularly partial to spraying fake tans on certain near-naked fellow female students. But given Adam/Isla/Annie's new identity, everyone accepted the transgender claim, not knowing this was someone with a pending rape case. Even with this new gender identity, applied as effortlessly as the spray tan solution, "Annie" had trouble fitting in with the other classmates, who recalled the student as a belligerent bully who showed a jealous streak when an attractive classmate practiced with others in the class.

At trial, Adam/Isla/Annie's defense attorney painted the brute as a potential victim if sent to prison. Perhaps that was the Scottish Prison Service's assumption, too, when initially housing him with women. After a public uproar, "Isla" was moved to a men's prison, but not before *Harry Potter* author J. K. Rowling got in a few digs at activists, including the Scottish First Minister, Nicola Sturgeon, who had been pushing to pass out so-called gender-recognition certificates with no wait time—just a simple declaration—that would allow anyone to be legally treated as the opposite sex. Rowling sarcastically tweeted: "Do you agree that a convicted double rapist who decided he was a woman after appearing in court belongs in a women's prison, or are you a nasty, far right bigot?"

Canada's prison system has been even more indulgent toward violent predators who prefer to bunk with women. Biological males who identify as transwomen are the ones who get to decide whether to serve their time in a men's or a women's prison. It wasn't until years after that policy was in place that the Correctional Service of Canada decided to do a study on this population's crimes. Quelle surprise! It found that 44 percent of its transwomen prisoners were sex offenders—and a whopping 94 percent of those hadn't discovered their inner oppressed trans identities until after they were caught. They committed their crimes as men, but entered their cells as transwomen. Those who claimed trans status were about twice as likely to have committed murder as other biological male inmates.

No one should be shocked that just four years after Canada's self-identification policy was put in place, the number of trans-identified inmates almost doubled.

But the above concerns other countries. Do we have any evidence that this is relevant to the United States? Unfortunately, yes.

President Donald Trump signed an Executive Order on January 20, 2025, that called for banning males from being housed in federal prisons for women (as of this writing, legal challenges to that order are pending). At the time he signed it, there were more than 1,500 men in federal prison who "identified" as women, though it's unclear how many of those men are locked into cells with women.

The federal Bureau of Prisons also doesn't report how many of these prisoners are intact males. What the bureau has revealed is that 48 percent of the men claiming female "identities" were sex offenders. (By contrast, sex offenders comprised only about 11 percent of the balance of the male prison population.)

President Trump's Executive Order, if ultimately upheld, can do nothing to protect women in state prisons. And that's where most of the country's prisoners are.

In September 2021, an Oregon man, Daniel Lee Smith, changed his name to Zera Lola Zombie, claimed to be trans, and said he was being discriminated against because he had been incarcerated in a males-only prison. Smith/Zombie is currently serving a thirty-five-year sentence for bludgeoning a girlfriend to death, and like "Isla Bryson," sports some rather prominent facial tattoos. The state transferred the aggrieved inmate to a women's prison. After three months, the state transferred Smith/Zombie back to the men's facility, and couldn't, or wouldn't, say why.

In one New Jersey women's prison, a female inmate described the number of male transfers into the facility as "obscene." Women prisoners complained that these intact biological males harassed them. But where did they all come from?

After an ACLU lawsuit, the prison was forced to transfer about two dozen biological males who identify as transwomen into the women-only prison. The first of these presumed transwomen transferees was Perry Cerf, who now goes by "Michelle" and was convicted of murdering a prostitute and drinking her blood. When another new trans-identified biological male physically attacked a female prisoner who had rejected a sexual advance, the biological male prisoner injured her badly enough for her to be hospitalized. The prison placed both the female victim and her trans attacker in solitary confinement.

At the same prison, two female inmates were impregnated by a couple of these "trans" inmates.

In 2023, the ACLU expressed outrage via tweet after Florida executed Duane Owen.

The focus of the organization's message wasn't an objection to the death penalty. Instead, its scathing statement concerned a matter closer to the current placement of the ACLU's heart. The tweet stated: "The state of Florida never provided medically necessary gender-affirming care to Duane Owen—causing her enormous suffering and violating her right to be free from cruel and unusual punishment for the more than 30 years she was in state custody."

Followers of the ACLU social media account might have learned nothing more about Owen than the cruel injustice recounted by the organization if it weren't for other readers who were able to quickly provide needed context in reply: "Duane stabbed 14-year-old Karen Slattery 18 times, killing her, then raped her corpse. He committed murder again years later."

A person convicted of murder and sentenced to die will use whatever strategies are available to go on living. And Owen apparently had.

He faked dementia (the inmate had a good memory according to prison mental health practitioners and had studied physics in prison). Psychiatrists for the state also claimed that he had faked schizophrenia, putting on a display of symptoms for their benefit, but showing no sign of the illness otherwise. They said much the same about his supposed gender confusion. He never presented himself as female. But all these disorders could be seen as mitigating factors in any appeal of his death sentence.

Owen's own confession called his gender claims into question.

During an interrogation in 1984, Owen said that he didn't know why he raped and murdered but he "liked to get away with things." He confessed to committing as many as five other murders and seven more rapes, but told a psychiatrist he would withhold information on those other crimes as leverage to delay his execution.

Later, at trial, when pleading insanity, he claimed that he raped and murdered because he needed to harvest women's hormones in order to become a woman.

When his lawyers appealed for leniency due to mental illness in 2002, the prosecutor claimed Owen had "studied up on sexual disorders and believed that the more crazy the story, the more people would believe he is crazy."

Identifying as trans, while not a "get-out-of-jail-free" card, is certainly a tactic that can make jail or prison somewhat less awful. If making that claim can get the ACLU to fervently stand up for you as if you were the victim, why wouldn't you do it? What would you have to lose?

Incels (heterosexual males who express anger about being involuntarily celibate) are portrayed by the Anti-Defamation League as hate group members—a brand of rightwing misogynist.

But put an involuntarily celibate male in high heels. Dab some bright red lipstick on that downturned mouth. Add some false eyelashes and a wig. Now, the incel is no longer a menace to society. He is a member of the oppressed and you must pour out your sympathy.

The penis of an incel in women's clothing is magically transformed into a female sex organ, or in the vernacular, a "girl dick."

No need to worry about whether the incel is a misogynist. Instead, that label applies to any lesbian who won't date an incel who claims that he, too, is a lesbian. Female-attracted women who don't consider such individuals to be members of their possible dating pools are told that they're expressing a "bigoted genital preference."

It's not that gender-confused incels are that much different from their brothers in involuntary celibacy. But they do have that ever-ready trans army behind them.

Carol, who you met in the first chapter, who for a few years thought of herself as trans until she said she realized, in her words, that being trans was "delusional," told me that she has run into a few of these natal males who call themselves both "transwomen" and "lesbians." She says that those who, like her, identified as trans, could blow off these male "lesbians" by claiming that sleeping with them would trigger their gender dysphoria.

"That was the only way you could get out of it," says Carol. "If you said any other thing, if you said, 'Well, no, I'm just not into males,' they'd answer, 'I'm not a male. How *dare* you?'"

According to Carol, it's been devastating, especially for the younger lesbians who've been indoctrinated into believing that a trans announcement makes a male instantly female. "I've sadly worked with a few young lesbians who are downright traumatized by the fact that they were pressured into sleeping with men," she says.

It can almost feel like the gay rights movement never happened. "We've all had to go underground again, precisely because men have completely infiltrated the lesbian community. And the LGBT community at large supports it." Support for inclusion of biological male "lesbians" in every space where actual lesbians gather and meet isn't solely coming from the LGBT community. "All of the dating apps, if you say that you are a lesbian and you only are interested in biological females, you will be kicked off the app."

In a Planet Fitness gym in Monroe, Georgia, where self-identification is the company policy, an intact male who claimed to be trans exposed himself to a nineteen-year-old female employee more than once. The gym did nothing about it. It wasn't until a customer came in with her fifteen-year-old niece and the guy who called himself trans decided to expose his buck-naked body, penis and all, to the teen, that police were called. They discovered that this "trans" character had a history of indecent exposure and a warrant out for arrest. As of October 12, 2023, Planet Fitness still had the following policy posted to its website: "Planet Fitness prohibits discrimination and harassment that is based on gender identity or gender expression in the workplace and in our clubs."

The fitness chain's management probably didn't believe there was any other option. The one fitness chain in the country that resisted allowing trans-identifying males in their formerly female-only locker rooms was sued by, you guessed it, the ACLU. (And in case you imagine I am a closet right-winger who has it in for the organization, I have an ACLU membership card in my wallet that expired a couple of years ago that reads: "Member since 2002." No, I won't be renewing.)

I want to be clear about something important. I've focused in this chapter on actual incidents of sexual violence and abuse of women and girls by males pretending to be female. But our privacy rights shouldn't hinge on whether any particular male poses a threat in female-only spaces.

When a male janitor gets ready to mop the floor in the girls' room at any school, anywhere, he first makes certain there are no girls still inside. That's not because otherwise, we assume he is going to assault any female he finds in there. It's because females' rights to privacy deserve to be respected.

We always knew this, and took it for granted, before the trans revolution. We understood that a strange male demanding to pee in the ladies room stall next to a girl doing the same was committing a de facto violation of her privacy, even if peeing is all he wanted to do. That's true even if he was wearing a dress and felt threatened by other males. Girls and women can't be forced to be human shields for fearful males.

The females for whom the restroom was designed aren't responsible for what a male chooses to wear, and they're not responsible for finding a solution to a male's dilemma as a result of his choices. Our rights cannot be made contingent on the choices and desires of the gender-confused.

I keep thinking of the chant you'll hear at any demonstration by trans activists:

Trans rights are human rights!
Trans rights are human rights!

And female rights are . . . what, exactly?

Chapter 10

Why Have We All Gone Mad?

"Men, it has been well said, think in herds; it will be seen that they go mad in herds, while they only recover their senses slowly, one by one."

—Charles MacKay, *Extraordinary Popular Delusions and the Madness of Crowds*

Leslie Eliot, an aspiring mental health counselor, was committed to the ideals of equality and justice. It didn't occur to her that what seemed like slight tweaks to the language—equity instead of equality; social justice instead of simply justice—signaled radical departures from her liberal views. But at the grad school she attended in Seattle, treating everyone equally was anathema. "Equity" meant people had to be treated differently, depending on their identities. So did "social justice."

A course syllabus included the following statement:

I acknowledge that racism, sexism, heterosexism, classism, ableism, ageism, nativism, and other forms of interpersonal and institutionalized forms of oppression exist. I will do my best to better understand my own privileged and marginalized identities and the power that these afford me.

195

That statement would eventually create a problem for her. She was told to restate that pledge in her own words and commit to it.

But she couldn't. Her principles wouldn't let her swear to beliefs that weren't true for her. Administrators informed her that her degree depended upon it. So, though she was only a few courses shy of meeting the requirements for graduation, she withdrew from the school.

As it turns out, it wouldn't have made much difference which school Leslie Elliot chose for her master's in social work. All accredited social work programs in the country now require that students share a critical social justice mindset that cannot be questioned.

But does this focus negatively affect how psychotherapy is practiced in the real world? David Habib Martin, LPC, a longtime psychotherapist and clinical supervisor in the state of Oregon, says it does.

Once students graduate, they spend another 1,900 hours under the guidance of more experienced mental health professionals like Habib Martin. And he sees confusion among these new graduates about the role of a therapist.

"It's backwards. You're not supposed to enter the therapy room with an already prepackaged idea of what's going on with your client," says Habib Martin. "And I'm noticing that with my supervisees that they don't know how to tell the difference between ethics and social justice work."

Even before they meet with a client, they're at a disadvantage because they've been trained to see "identities" rather than just individuals in need of help. Habib Martin is often sought out as a supervisor by other men entering the counseling field, and their training tells them that males, especially white heterosexual ones, are privileged and their masculinity is toxic. "They've been told all during their grad school that their voice needs to take a back seat. And now they're entering the therapy room and they're like, 'What do I say to people?' They're like, 'I'm a straight white guy. Should I be doing this job?'"

When indoctrination tells therapists that "identity" matters more than anything else, that translates into a disadvantage for any clients they see.

"They tell you the job is to be an activist no matter what you're doing," explains Habib Martin. "And that is the antithesis of therapeutic because you're no longer client centered. You can't be."

If such an ideology is injected into every aspect of the social work curriculum, it makes more sense that so many therapists are open to "affirming" trans identities in children.

But critical social justice ideology also influences the English curriculum and the philosophy curriculum. In medical school, tomorrow's doctors are required to take courses in "social justice" that, by now, you can guess, are mislabeled. Math? Yes, there too.

At Vanderbilt University's Peabody College of Education and Human Development, Luis Antonio Leyva, an assistant professor, "discovered" that math instruction was somehow transphobic.

Leyva was taken seriously enough that he got to present his ideas at the Joint Mathematics Meetings in Boston, Massachusetts, in 2023, billed as the largest mathematics gathering in the world. His presentation, according to the program, was titled: "Undergraduate Mathematics Education as a White, Cisheteropatriarchal Space and Opportunities for Structural Disruption to Advance Queer of Color Justice."

Here, in part, is how he described his presentation:

Findings depict how Black, Latin, and Asian [queer and transgender] students' narratives of experience reflect forms of intersectionality, or instances of oppression and resistance at intersecting systems of white supremacy and cisheteropatriarchy (or white cisheteropatriarchy).

Did you get all that? Right. Neither did I. But the newly minted math teachers he trains will deliver this "wisdom" wherever they end up teaching.

A 2021 article in *School Library Journal* complained that Shakespeare's works were "full of problematic, outdated ideas." Well, he was born in the sixteenth century, so a few outdated ideas are to be expected, but it also accused the man considered the greatest English language playwright to ever have lived of bigotry, sexism, and classism. The piece quoted several teachers who had decided they'd had enough of the "white, cisgender, heterosexual" bard and stated that they wouldn't be subjecting their students to any further lessons in his works.

Meanwhile, at Shakespeare's Globe Theatre in London, England, Joan of Arc was portrayed as non-binary in a recent play, complete with they/them pronouns. Around the same time, an academic, writing for the Globe Theatre's in-house publication, claimed that Queen Elizabeth I and tenth century Queen Aethelflaed of the Mercians were both transgender, because each woman had led armies.

Biology textbooks, too, now claim that sex isn't quite so settled. According to the high school textbook *Experience Biology*, published by Savvas Learning Company, just because your anatomy pegged you as either male or female, that didn't resolve the issue. No, say the book's authors, sex is more complicated than that. What if your anatomy doesn't match your inner sense of your own gender? (Note to the authors of *Experience Biology*: whatever you imagine you're teaching, it isn't biology).

And an AP biology textbook *Biology in Focus* published by Pearson claimed that 1 percent of all babies are born intersex (wildly untrue; the actual figure is only 0.018 percent of all births, which is more than an order of magnitude fewer) and that sex is "assigned" at birth rather than observed. It also teaches kids that a person might "have an assigned sex of female but a male gender identity."

This is not biology. It's ideology.

The state of affairs over in anthropology is no better. The organizers of the September 2023 American Anthropological Association conference canceled a panel for their program titled "Let's Talk about Sex Baby: Why Biological Sex Remains a Necessary Analytic Category in Anthropology."

The letter sent to the canceled panelists explained: "The reason the session deserved further scrutiny was that the ideas were advanced in such a way as to cause harm to members represented by the Trans and LGBTQI of the anthropological community as well as the community at large."

In anthropology, too, sex is out. Gender is in.

The head of the American Library Association has advocated for "queering the catalogue."

And there are places in the world, including Spain, Mexico, the United Kingdom, and even New York City, where you're at risk of legal peril for "misgendering" someone (i.e., correctly identifying their sex).

Teddy Cook, an Australian woman who identifies as a man, is a perfect example of what Gayle Rubin labeled an oppressed sexual minority in her manifesto that launched the queer theory movement. Cook begged for understanding and acceptance at a meeting of the Australian parliament when speaking passionately against a proposed law that would have banned lessons in gender ideology in that country's schools. She insisted that people like her "... *are not powerful enough to disrupt the culture of this country. Many of us, even though we are incredibly resilient, are just trying to get through the day, really. We are not the threat you imagine us to be.*"

All Cook was asking for, she claimed, was some dignity. She got accolades for that speech. In 2023, the World Health Organization (WHO) chose her to join a panel of about twenty health experts from around the world who would help develop guidelines for transgender health care. It didn't appear to matter that Cook's social media posts were, according to a *Daily Mail* article, "awash with X-rated material, including public nudity, bondage parties, trans orgies and even a photo of a man apparently having sex with a dog."

Most of those who fall into one of Rubin's "sexual minorities" categories aren't just exhibiting a few harmless quirks. If publicly displaying pornographic images, including bestiality, didn't disqualify Teddy Cook from a high-profile position with an organization like the WHO, then quite clearly, widespread acceptance of queer theory *is* powerful enough to disrupt the culture.

So the question becomes, is this what we want for our children? For ourselves?

Where *should* we draw the line? We're approaching a place where all lines must be erased lest those drawing them risk being shunned as transphobes, prudes, and bigots who are cruelly discriminating against an oppressed minority.

Again, is this what we want?

Earlier in my research, I was skeptical of the notion that children were being sexually "groomed" by proponents of queer theory. Sure, the document that originally linked "sexual minorities" to social justice spilled a ton of ink justifying the obliteration of sexual boundaries, including those that prohibit adult sex with children. But that didn't mean that this had any relevance to what was happening in schools today. There's theory and then there's practice, and they're different. That's what I assumed at the time.

Let me share the evidence that changed my mind.

In early 2022, I was researching critical race theory, which, along with queer theory, is the other main branch of critical social justice ideology. White people were falling all over themselves discussing their attempts to be "less white," trying to outdo other white people in their complaints about how awful white people were.

I found it outlandish and planned to write about it. I was also looking into the trans craze, but was initially narrowly focused on the colossal increase in teen girls who had suddenly and inexplicably declared themselves to be boys.

On Twitter, I followed the conservative firebrand Chris Rufo because he'd been documenting critical race theory–related incidents.

One day in the summer of 2022, Rufo posted something about Portland Public Schools' sex education curriculum for little kids. It was so outrageous, I knew (or believed at the time that I knew) that it couldn't be true.

In a file attached to his post, Rufo presented what he said were sex education curriculum documents. He claimed these materials had originated from Portland—some directed at kindergarten through third graders—and had been leaked to him. But he had no evidence to show that their reported provenance was genuine.

Among the images in the curriculum materials were illustrations of two nude children, a boy and a girl. The boy was first shown standing. Next to that illustration were close-up images of his genitals with his thighs spread wide. A line from each body part led to text: penis, scrotum, testicles, urethra opening, anus.

On the next page was a nude girl, first standing as the boy had been, and then, the extreme close-up of her genitals between her thighs, which, like the boy's, were spread wide. This is roughly the view a gynecologist would have when a girl or woman is on her back and her feet are in stirrups. As with the boy, there was a line to each part of the genital anatomy and a label: vulva, clitoris outside, urethra opening, vagina opening, anus.

These illustrations were extremely explicit.

I live close to Portland, so I emailed members of my weekly discussion group, one of whom had been a city manager in a small city in the same county as Portland, and another who was deeply involved with local charities. These were knowledgeable, connected people. If kids were being shown such explicit images, they or someone they knew would have heard, or so I assumed. I asked if anyone knew parents or teachers in the school system who could confirm the report.

No one could. Nor could I find any reference to such materials or lessons on the Portland Public Schools website. I read through the state's statutory mandates and the materials Rufo posted didn't appear to meet those.

But just to be sure, I emailed Portland Public Schools, with the link to Rufo's purported kindergarten sex ed materials, and asked: "Please let me know if this is an actual PPS curriculum document."

I got a friendly reply from a media rep from the school system about a week later: "PPS is aware that there is misinformation regarding our sexuality education classes in the media space. The slide deck that is circulating in the media is not property of PPS."

Confident that the school's response meant Rufo was misinformed, I tweeted that I'd heard from Portland Public Schools and the purported sex ed document was not theirs.

Since then, I've interviewed countless parents and experts and looked into what's been happening in schools across the nation. Part of my research has involved watching videos of angry parents at school board meetings, demanding that middle school libraries not stock their shelves with porn. And yes, at least a dozen books that some schools happily supply to children in elementary, middle, and high school are graphic enough to be called porn.

Mainstream news media has reported unprecedented attempts to ban books. Typically, the stories suggest that crazed rightwing parents are trying to pull beloved tales like *To Kill a Mockingbird*, *Catcher in the*

Rye, and *Of Mice and Men* off the shelves. As I write this, Change.org has twenty-six petitions you can sign to protest book banning.

Granted, there are parents who oppose exposing their children to books like *To Kill a Mockingbird.* But there's a whole different list of books that would never have made it into a school library a decade ago because of the explicit sexual images and text. And those are being opposed by a whole different contingent of parents, including moms and dads who probably would be thrilled if their kids took the time to read *To Kill a Mockingbird.*

If liberal and moderate parents understood that X-rated material appeared in some of the books that await kids in school libraries around the country, instead of signing petitions against book bans, many probably would be lodging protests against offering porn to children.

Parents and others have tried to read from lewd children's books at school board meetings across the country to demonstrate the problem. But school board officials almost always order them to stop. That's because the one thing everyone agrees upon is that certain passages from these challenged kids' books are obscene. And no one is permitted to use obscene language at school board meetings. Here's a small sample:

> *I put some lube on [the condom] and got him up on his knees and I began to slide into him from behind.* (All Boys Aren't Blue)

> *From six up, I used to kiss other guys in my neighborhood, make out with them, and perform oral sex on them. I liked it.* (Beyond Magenta)

> *I can't wait to have your cock in my mouth. I'm going to give you the blowjob of your life.* (Gender Queer)

> *There is only one hard and fast rule when it comes to blow jobs— WATCH THE TEETH.* (This Book Is Gay)

You get the idea.

A dad shared a photo with me that he took of a poster in his son's middle school that promoted a number of challenged books, including all four of the above. The poster asked kids for their reaction to attempts to ban the titles. Just tell a teen, *your parents don't want you to read this*, and you can bet there will be a waiting list for the title at the library. Other books that parents have asked to have removed from children's libraries include one called *Let's Talk about It*, which tells kids to go on the internet to "to research fantasies and kinks," because they'll find lots of helpful people there with the same interests.

Well, of course, they will. Those "helpful" people are known as groomers if not pedophiles.

Other school library books that alarmed parents had illustrations of naked people having sex, gay and straight.

There was a time, not long ago, when an adult would have been brought up on charges if he or she provided a minor with such reading material.

Even so, not every child reads every library book. But if sexually explicit books or other materials are used to teach classes, all the children in the class are exposed.

Imagine sitting in a room full of your peers—a room you can't easily leave without causing a stir. All the people in the room are being surveyed about how comfortable they are with certain sexual acts.

Here's one of the questions:

Are you:
Not comfortable, somewhat comfortable, or very comfortable masturbating in the same room (with another person)?

Here's another one:

Are you:
Not comfortable, somewhat comfortable, or very comfortable with anal sex?

Now imagine you're a fifteen-year-old. Because that's how old you'd be if you were in that room being asked those questions.

The survey is part of the sex education curriculum in a San Francisco–area school district. This particular course is based on "Be Real,

Be Ready," published by the Adolescent Health Working Group. But similar materials might be found in the sex ed classes in almost any school with a liberal or progressive bent. The curriculum also covers a wide range of other sex acts: dry humping; oral sex; using the fingers and hand to stroke or massage another's genitals; and vaginal intercourse.

Some parents who learned what their kids were being asked about were appalled. One dad wrote to the superintendent of the school district demanding to know why the school was asking kids about their comfort level with masturbating around others and anal sex. The superintendent responded that the questions were meant to help kids understand consent. But that doesn't actually make any sense. No teacher needs to discuss the full menu of all possible sex acts that someone might propose to a kid in order to let them know they have the right to say no.

Lisa Mullins' daughter was a sophomore in the school district that asked kids about their comfort levels with various sex acts. At the time, Mullins had no reason to suspect that sex ed had changed so radically from when she was a teen. Then she overheard her daughter's teacher lecturing students in a Zoom class during the Covid lockdown. The first thing that caught her attention was a discussion about the "gender unicorn," which is used to tell kids that their sex and gender might not match. From there, she overheard talk of anal sex, and "lube, lube, lube," along with misinformation about basic sexual anatomy.

It angered Mullins that her fifteen-year-old daughter was being exposed to complete nonsense. So she visited the Adolescent Health Working Group's website to review some of the curriculum materials used. There, she discovered a page titled "Healthy Relationships" that listed "Friends with Benefits," "Polyamorous," "Hook-up," and other non-monogamous sexual escapades under that "Healthy" title.

Why was the school teaching this? It not only went against the morals she and her husband had tried to instill in their children but also had no educational value at all.

As wildly inappropriate as these lessons were, they were being given in high school. They could be destabilizing for certain students, but not to the degree that explicit material would be to younger children.

The first solid evidence I found that not just transgender but hyper-sexualized material was being taught in elementary school classrooms came from Alesha Perkins, the Olympia, Washington, mom you met in an earlier chapter.

A parent forwarded a pamphlet to Alesha that had formed the basis of a fourth-grade lesson that was supposed to be about puberty. The pamphlets were provided by Planned Parenthood's Teen Council (Planned Parenthood is the single largest provider in the United States of sex ed materials). The pages, as you might expect, were filled with trans propaganda. For example, a "gender wheel" suggested to children that they turn it to choose their new gender and pronouns. But also included was something that no one, not even parents inured to constant trans indoctrination, could have anticipated:

- A two-page full-color spread consisting entirely of illustrations of human genitalia;
- Fifteen explicit illustrations of male genitals;
- Thirty explicit pictures of female genitals;
- Thirteen intersex genital images.

One of the images showed a woman's pubic hair styled in the form of a cat's face. In two others, the pubic hair was shaved into heart shapes.

What purpose might there be in distributing such materials to nine- and ten-year-old children?

The pamphlet also included an image of puberty blockers under the heading: "Supplies That Could Be Helpful During Puberty!"

That was when I thought back to Rufo's post.

Had I been too quick to assume that I'd gotten a straight answer from the Portland Public Schools' media contact?

I placed a public records request with Portland schools for any and all materials related to the sex ed curriculum for grades K–8, including teacher's guidelines.

About six weeks later, I got an email with a single link. The link would take me to an "overview of district-wide K–12 Health Curriculum."

The email was signed by a different media person than the one I'd heard from two years earlier and, of course, included his pronouns.

I clicked the link, not expecting much.

Now, I wonder if he/him/his even knew what was at that link. Right there, among the overview documents, were a few of the same images that Rufo had had leaked to him in 2022. The text had since been revised. The earlier text stated, "A lot of times people with these parts are girls, but any gender and kid can have any type of body."

In the newer version, the words "girls" and "boys" had been replaced with "person with a vulva" and "person with a penis," respectively. The teacher's guide explained that words like boy and girl were being removed to show support for transgender and non-binary students.

The materials stated that the lesson was for kids in kindergarten through third grade and were "**developmentally appropriate**." [emphasis added].

This, right here, is sort of a Jedi mind trick, meant to blunt the concerns of any parents who wonder why their children are being introduced to such materials. *"Nothing to see here, folks. It's all 'developmentally appropriate.'"*

But who decided that? What research did they use to determine that these claims of developmental appropriateness were valid?

I filed a new public records request for "any and all documents related to the criteria Portland Schools uses to determine that sexual education materials for K–5 are developmentally appropriate for the age groups taught." I got a several-week runaround. He/him/his couldn't provide any documents that showed how or if these images were determined to be developmentally appropriate. That's probably because they simply aren't.

Though I found documentation showing that Planned Parenthood's Teen Council had supplied some sex ed materials to Portland, I couldn't get access to those documents, so I wasn't able to determine if they were the same as the ones used in Olympia.

The documents I was allowed to access were broken out by grade. In kindergarten and first grade, the standing images of the nude boy and girl were shown and the "person with a penis" had circumcised and uncircumcised versions. By second grade, kids were being taught about the sensitivity of the clitoris while examining close-up explicit illustrations—thighs spread wide—of children's genitals.

Think about that for a moment. What's the educational value for a child that young?

If there's no discernible educational value, what's the objective, other than to destabilize a child's boundaries?

And whose agenda does that serve?

A favorite party game for little kids like the second graders being shown these images is "pin the tail on the donkey." The lesson plan for teachers presenting the materials is similar, except that now it's "pin the label on the clitoris."

Teachers are told to have kids participate in the lesson by placing sticky note labels on the images of parts of the sexual anatomy between those widely spread thighs. Oh, and the lesson is labeled: *"Understanding Our Bodies Unit 4: Growth and Development + Violence Prevention 2nd Grade Content."*

Like the Olympia schools' "puberty" lesson with its explicit genital images, Portland's "violence prevention" lesson is sexualizing little kids by stealth, violating any boundaries that their parents might have set in place.

The teachers tasked with presenting these materials are just teaching what they're told to. The vast majority almost certainly have no such agenda.

But someone does. Someone wrote these materials. Someone illustrated them. Someone decided how teachers should talk to children about them. And someone published them.

Of course, no lesson in sex ed for tiny tykes would be complete without confusing the kids about what sex they actually are. A section from the first grade teacher's guide on "gender identity" helps teachers explain to first graders that just because they have boy or girl body parts, that doesn't make them boys and girls. They might feel like the opposite sex, or *"you might not feel like you're a boy or a girl, but you're a little bit of both."*

Another part of the **first grade** teacher's guide includes a description of the vaginal canal, describing its shape and size, and including this:

*The vagina has great elasticity, **and can adjust to the size of a penis**
. . .* [emphasis added]

The guide states that it's up to the first-grade teacher to decide how much of this to share with students "in ways that are age appropriate."

How can it possibly be age appropriate *at all*, no matter how a teacher presents information, to discuss—**in the first grade**—the vagina's ability to adjust to the size of a penis?

The hyper-sexualization of school children isn't exclusively a US problem. *Reduxx* magazine has reported on a number of troubling incidents in other countries, as well. For example, an Austrian kindergarten displayed large posters of people taking showers. One depicted a nude man who presumably identified as a woman; he had both a penis and breasts. Another showed a naked obese man showering with a young boy. A third displayed a nude adult male showering with two nude children, a little girl and boy. The caption accompanying the images was translated by the magazine as "Bodies naked and bare, vulva, penis, breasts, butts. You decide for yourself, indeed! Bodies are cool!" The parents of two kindergarteners complained that such images were inappropriate for little ones and requested that they be removed.

Instead, the school expelled the children of the parents who complained, insisting that children aged one to six years old needed such sex education.

And in Taiwan, a private school asked fourteen- and fifteen-year-old students to complete a survey with questions such as:

Have you ever taken nude or sexually explicit pictures of yourself?

Have you had sexual intercourse? (Penile, vaginal, or anal penetration)

Have you ever sexted?

None of this passes the "ick" test.

How on Earth did we let this happen?

"What you're asking really is, how does a mass psychosis take over a society?"

Derrick Jensen is one of the more insightful people I've interviewed for this book. So, yes, I was asking him to help me figure this out: how did a mass psychogenic illness, or as he put it more bluntly, a mass psychosis, migrate from the dark corners of the university to overtake primary school systems of the United States, Canada, the United Kingdom, and virtually every other industrialized country of the so-called First World?

Why have we all gone mad?

I first encountered Jensen when I stumbled upon his brilliant takedown, "Queer Theory Jeopardy." In a video that went viral, he demonstrated that children have always been targets of queer theorists, and not just as belief-system recruits.

One of the founders of Deep Green Resistance and dubbed by *Democracy Now!* the poet-philosopher of the ecological movement, Jensen focuses most of his energy on the fight to preserve wild beings and wild places. But the prolific author has also written several books about history, culture, and society. He'd been beloved by people on what used to be the far left. Then he decided to write about the left's most extreme edge: anything-goes anarchism.

Jensen is in sync with what he calls the sane anarchist's point of view: that because governments take better care of corporations than they do of people, cooperation within communities has more potential to attend to the needs of community members than do central governments. But he has a problem with anarchism's less sane and more dominant branch. That branch argues that because those in power make laws that benefit the powerful, all laws and all social rules are inherently oppressive.

"And they mean *all*. And so I'm looking into this, and I'm like, okay, what about pedophilia?"

What he found was that notable anarchists also considered restrictions against sex with children oppressive. And having decided that any restrictions against pedophilia were inherently oppressive, certain anarchists had actively advocated for breaking down *all* barriers to adults having sex with children.

"The biggest anarchist magazine put out an entire issue devoted to promoting pedophilia," he says. "Benjamin Tucker, one of the most famous American anarchists 120 years ago, promoted pedophilia. John Henry Mackie, one of the most famous anarchists in Europe in the 1910s and 1920s, he wrote a whole series of books about how important it is to be able to rape children. And so, there's a long connection there."

But what does any of this have to do with postmodernism, queer theory, and the trans craze among kids?

You'll recall that queer theory *also* promotes the belief that all rules related to sex are inherently oppressive. Given the agreement on that point, it's not surprising that the current day anarchist movement is allied with gender ideology—or that influential queer theorists share the view that sexualizing children actually liberates children.

Looking into one movement's perverse instincts led Jensen to probe more deeply into the other's.

"Queer theory . . . asks a really good question, which is: how do certain things become normal? And especially sexual things. That's a really focused question. That's a great question," says Jensen. "How did the wage economy become normalized? How did capitalism become normalized? How did driving on the right side of the road become normalized? Fascinating question. For sex, why is homosexuality stigmatized? Good question."

But, he says, queer theory answered the question about how sexual things become normalized in the stupidest way possible.

"Because strictures against homosexuality are oppressive and harmful, therefore, all strictures against all forms of sex are oppressive and harmful . . . I still can't believe how popular, I mean, how much it controls discourse, when it is so vile."

Most people who support gender ideology claim—and probably believe—that it has nothing to do with the sexualization of children. They might not know that a celebrity trans activist recently pooh-poohed concerns about males in girls' bathrooms with this: "These days, the narrative is that transgender people will come into bathrooms and abuse little girls . . . Little girls are also kinky. Your kids aren't as straight and narrow as you think."

Jensen was understandably disturbed by what he'd discovered about queer theory's attitudes toward sexualizing children. So he included a chapter about it in the book he'd been working on, *Anarchism and the Politics of Violation.* The book was due to be published sometime in late 2018 or early 2019.

Because of the queer theory chapter, "The publisher held it for five years and then severed their relationship with me," Jensen says. (As of this writing, Amazon still lists *Anarchism and the Politics of Violation,* with an expected publication date of January 2, 2079. This date is not a typo.)

Another Jensen book, *Bright Green Lies*, was canceled by a separate publisher, due to Jensen's and his co-authors' opposition to gender ideology. The subject matter of *Bright Green Lies* has nothing to do with gender or queer theory or its relationship to pedophilia. Instead, the book marked a return to Jensen's primary focus: how industrialization is killing the planet, and why wind and solar technology won't save it.

Publishers weren't just canceling his books. They were canceling Derrick Jensen.

This wasn't the first time Jensen had angered gender ideologues, but it was the most consequential for his writing career. Several years prior, a male who identified as a woman wrote to him, asking to attend a conference that was being held by Deep Green Resistance. Female members of the group told Jensen that they didn't want to bunk with a male, no matter how he identified. So, Jensen told the trans-identifying male that it would be fine for him to attend but he would be housed with other males. And they wouldn't call him "she."

"And he immediately wrote back and said, 'I hope you die from disease,' then publicized it. And within days, I was receiving a lot of death threats. The women in [Deep Green Resistance] were receiving rape and death threats. People were saying that they were going to rape and murder the women's children. So that was really my introduction to the discourse surrounding that issue."

For expressing "incorrect" views, the far left eco-warrior has also been disinvited from speaking to environmental group gatherings, and from speaking to students and faculty at universities.

Derrick Jensen was particularly appalled by Gayle Rubin's *Thinking Sex*. "About half of it's an apology for pedophilia. It's completely nuts."

But if Jensen was simply highlighting the stated positions of the author of queer theory's founding document, the people who inspired her writing, and numerous subsequent proponents, why should those who embrace queer theory have a problem with Jensen noticing what they stand for?

Jensen thinks it's because his detractors didn't understand what they thought they were defending.

"They're saying nobody gets to complain about queer theory. But they've never read it."

That's one of the more peculiar things about queer theory. Somehow, as it filtered into the larger culture, the pedophilic references have gotten sanitized out of it. But as illustrated by the highly sexualized materials being used to teach children in the earliest grades, that doesn't mean those concepts aren't still operative.

The social justice façade converts the underlying theme of transgressive sex into a heroic tale of dismantling oppression. Somehow it's worked. Relatively few parents and teachers have revolted, considering what's being promoted. A startling number seem to believe they are heroes for actively participating.

Because he's studied queer theory with a skeptical eye for more than a decade, I was confident Jensen would have insights into how this patently ridiculous, and to use his word, "vile" ideology became the basis of so many rules and laws that we're increasingly forced to live by. But Jensen was stumped. We chewed over what might be responsible.

"In terms of this taking over everything, it doesn't hurt that the Pritzkers have billions of dollars," he said.

The Pritzker family that Jensen referred to, heirs to the Hyatt Hotels fortune, includes not only Jennifer Pritzker, who was originally named James, but also the presumably autogynephilic male's cousins, one of whom is, as I write this, the governor of Illinois. Jennifer Pritzker served as a colonel in the Army National Guard. Married twice, he fathered one child with one wife and two with another, then announced that he was trans in 2013 at the age of sixty-three. Pritzker has been presenting himself as a woman since.

Journalist Jennifer Bilek has written at length about how Jennifer has poured millions into pushing the transgender cause and how other members of the Pritzker family have helped to push the ideology. Bilek's piece in *Tablet* magazine laid out how Jennifer Pritzker, through his Tawani Foundation, funded a who's who of organizations involved in promoting transgenderism, including the Human Rights Campaign (HRC), the Williams Institute, the National Center for Transgender Equality, the Transgender Legal Defense and Education Fund, the American Civil Liberties Union (ACLU), and the World Professional Association of Transgender Health.

Bilek's reporting provides a plausible reason for why so much of the ACLU's energy now goes toward fighting to eliminate biological female-only spaces so that males who claim to be female have access. That mission now appears to consume at least as much of the ACLU's energy as protecting free expression (which is what the organization had previously been best known for). It also might help explain how the HRC was able to reinvent itself. HRC had been the driving force behind the legalization of gay marriage in the United States. It didn't seem to have as much reason to exist once that campaign succeeded. Thanks in part to Pritzker money, it's now a very successful "trans rights" group.

But does money alone, even barrels of it, ensure public acceptance of the ideas being promoted? The entire Pritzker family fortune is estimated to be $36.9 billion. Jennifer's share of that is estimated at $1.9 billion. That's serious capital, but is whatever portion Pritzker uses to prop up and promote the ideology enough to produce and sustain a mass psychogenic event that spans the industrialized world?

How much money would it take to evaporate the skepticism and critical thinking skills of countless seemingly intelligent people, not just in education but also in media, the medical profession, the mental health field, state and federal governments, and nonprofit organizations? A persuasive public relations campaign can sway public opinion, but when the truth dribbles out, as it has, in a multitude of ways, what keeps all those believers in the fold?

Bilek's research into Jennifer Pritzker's investment is interesting information. I've no doubt that his donations to transgender-promoting organizations have had an effect. But I'm not persuaded that one guy, or even one family, whatever their net worth, could have quite as profound an influence as Bilek believes.

I did some digging of my own, and while it's impossible to account for all the money that goes toward promoting trans ideology, it's probably not as massive a war chest as Bilek suggests. Nor is it all coming from Pritzker and his allies.

The majority of the rainbows-and-unicorns transgenderism promotion has been done for free by virtually every major media organization, a good chunk of the entertainment industry, almost all medical associations, almost every liberal college and university, every liberal and progressive K–12 public school system, and most so-called progressive political figures. While Jennifer Pritzker's donations to nonprofits promoting transgenderism like the ACLU, the HRC, and others increased their reach, and their ability to influence all the other figures propping up the ideology, the effect has been far greater than what the actual donation amounts suggest would be possible.

And that's just in this country. It's more or less the same story in the rest of the Western world. To buy this kind of influence for any other cause would likely wipe out the entire Pritzker family fortune in a year.

That's not to say no one is making money on transgenderism. The average cost of a vaginoplasty in 2019 was $53,645, and for phalloplasty, it was $133,911. The average cost of cross-sex hormones, according to one mail order supplier, is from $80 to $95 per month. That adds up when it's every month for the rest of a young person's life.

And yet, you can't explain this phenomenon simply by counting up the cash.

In the eighteen months or so since Derrick Jensen and I discussed it, I've spent countless hours pondering the question: how did so many different people and organizations buy into and help sustain the trans craze, despite the abject absurdity of it all, despite its destructiveness, despite its contradicting (with zero evidence) almost everything about sex that we know to be true? I've examined all the theories and looked into all the groups that have been singled out by other journalists and authors, and I've concluded that it's not any single group or individual or idea or incentive.

It's all of them.

Gender ideology is bolstered and held together by a web of unlikely allies: the wealthy transvestic fetishists and autogynephiles; the indoctrinated educators; the established nonprofits seeking new sources of revenue; the moms and dads who've "affirmed" their children and desperately need for it to have been the right call; the medical and mental health professionals profiting from trans-related services; the kids who've been purposely confused by their elders; the gays and lesbians who see the T as part of their tribe; the college-educated social justice warriors; all the other "sexual minorities," including the most perverted, demanding understanding and acceptance; the legacy media that report trans insanity as if it were Truth itself; and the army of virtue signalers whose interest is almost entirely based on a narcissistic desire for high fives and attaboys.

Only such a grotesquely idiosyncratic coalition could keep the madness going for as long as it has, across thousands of miles and more than a dozen countries.

In the next chapter, we'll consider what the rest of us need to do if we hope to counter this unlikely coalition's effects.

Chapter 11

It's Time to Reclaim
Reality and Sanity

*"If you can keep your head when all about you
Are losing theirs and blaming it on you . . ."*

—Rudyard Kipling

In *Thinking Sex*, Gayle Rubin condemned society's fear of the sexual deviant and ridiculed the concern that "the barrier against scary sex will crumble and something unspeakable will skitter across."

In much the same way, almost forty years later, Teddy Cook shamed the Australian parliament into backing off the notion that sexual deviants, who constitute only a minority of the population, could disrupt an entire culture.

And yet, what each dismissed is now our reality.

In his 1929 book *The Thing*, G. K. Chesterton wrote of a hypothetical situation where a reformer comes upon an obstacle, a fence, for example, that doesn't seem to be serving any purpose. The reformer wants to knock it down, but Chesterton advises against even considering its removal before the person bent on dismantling it understands why it was erected in the first place. It was built for a reason. And you can't determine what you'll be allowing to cross that boundary if you take it down without knowing the reason.

Our tolerant society demolished what we assumed was an unnecessary fence because the people on the other side told us it hurt them not to be able to pass freely. *Be kind*, they said. That was all it took. We didn't see that that boundary served any purpose. And because we failed to understand why it was there, we couldn't begin to imagine what might come through once we dismantled it.

Look at what's skittered out now that, in some instances, we've largely agreed to erase the line between male and female.

Notice that we haven't actually lessened the number of barriers we live with. Instead, we've erected new barriers, ones that restrain free thought, movement, and speech, and also constrain us from safeguarding the vulnerable.

We're so intimidated by these new barriers, we avoid speaking truthfully about which sexes humans are capable of being. We suppress our natural instincts to protect young people from what skitters across that line Rubin wrote about, because we're not allowed to notice that any of it is dangerous. Some of the new barriers have been written into laws that make the acknowledgment of sexual reality illegal. It often seems that anything or anyone, once wrapped in rainbow colors, becomes impervious to previous norms.

Consider, for example, a video recently posted on X (formerly Twitter), of a guy walking down a busy street in Seattle wearing hiking boots and thigh-high rainbow legwarmers. Nothing else. The naked guy's long straight brown hair fell halfway to his waist. He sported bouncy smallish breasts (I'd guess an A cup), almost certainly due to taking cross-sex hormones. His penis, fully erect, jutted perpendicular to the rest of him as he strode along. Commenters on X and Reddit wrote that this guy had been exposing himself around their Capitol Hill neighborhood for quite some time. As far as anyone knew, he'd never been arrested for it.

If he were wearing a trench coat and only randomly flashing passersby, would cops have hauled him in? My guess is yes. My guess is that as long as he wraps some part of himself in rainbow colors, he can expose the rest to everyone he passes, and no one will dare say a word.

In a middle school in another part of Washington state, instead of giving the sex ed lesson that was an approved part of the curriculum, a science teacher set up a projector screen, Googled images of "penises and vaginas," and told kids to sketch what they saw. One girl who was in that class said that the images that came up in the search were so shocking, she needed counseling after the class. If this had happened a decade or so previously, that teacher almost certainly would have been fired. But the teacher runs the school's GSA club. Those rainbow colors act like an invisible shield. Is anyone surprised that, despite complaints, she's still teaching the same classes in the same school?

In Indiana, a man with tattoos covering his face, currently serving a fifty-five-year sentence for murdering his eleven-month-old stepdaughter, claimed to identify as a Muslim, Wiccan woman. When the state declined to cover his genital surgery, the ACLU sued. A federal judge ruled that his surgery is medically necessary and the state must pay for it.

Across the thresholds of all the torn-down fences, utter madness is skittering past. And it's happening in Western societies everywhere, not just in the United States.

In Victoria, Australia, parents risk up to a ten-year prison sentence if they suppress their children's attempts to get puberty blockers, or cross-sex hormones, or mutilating trans surgeries—or if they even attempt to talk their kids out of the idea that they were born in the wrong body. Parents also risk prosecution if they take their kids out of Victoria to avoid compliance. The law actually expressly forbids so much as praying that the kids will accept reality.

In England, in the town of Blaydon, an "adult nursery" (for adults with diaper fetishes who identify as babies and toddlers) has been approved for a business license according to British detransitioner Ritchie Herron. It's unclear whether the nursery's workers will change those adult diapers when soiled and clean the fetishists' bottoms, or whether other kinksters are expected to volunteer for the job.

In the south of France, a gynecologist had his license to practice suspended because the doctor told a man who identified as female that, as a gynecologist, he was only qualified to examine women. Further north, in Paris, the fashion house Balenciaga made a splash running ads featuring children hugging teddy bears outfitted with fetish gear.

In Scotland, at Edinburgh Napier University, midwifery students were taught how to care for a "birthing person" with a penis and scrotum. Curricular materials actually claimed "that biological males can get pregnant and give birth through their penis," according to documents leaked to *Reduxx* magazine from the school.

In Spain, according to the same magazine, a man who identifies as a woman was sentenced to six months in prison because he made "transphobic" remarks about another man who identifies as a woman.

In Canada, a proposed amendment to its Human Rights Act, called the Online Harms Act, would label some social media comments regarding "gender identity or expression" crimes if, by some murky standard, officials decided the comments were motivated by hate. "The new offence would carry a maximum punishment of **imprisonment for life.**" [emphasis added].

Is it possible to repair and fortify the fences we've torn apart now that we know what's on the other side?

And how can we help those who bought into the belief system and had irreparable damage done to their bodies?

When Hannah Ulery escaped from the cult she'd grown up in, she was forced to leave her parents and brother behind. Both while in the cult and after her escape, she'd been raped and molested. She suffered from a host of extreme mental health issues: OCD, ADHD, bipolar disorder with psychosis, major depression, anxiety, and body dysmorphia. She also had dissociative identity disorder, formerly known as multiple personality disorder. Her traumatized psyche had fragmented into a multitude of alter egos.

By any standards, Hannah Ulery was mentally disabled. No one in her condition would be capable of informed consent.

But the therapist who treated her pushed her to identify as a male after learning that Hannah was a lesbian and that a few of Hannah's "alters" were male. Hannah at first resisted the suggestion to take testosterone, but eventually acquiesced. Her doctors knew she was unable at times to distinguish reality from fantasy. They knew that one of her alternate personalities was dead set against taking testosterone and attempted to sabotage the doctors' "treatment." They prescribed the cross-sex hormone to her anyway.

Years later, Hannah, who has since changed her name to Layton, moved to North Carolina, where she got the kind of psychotherapy she'd always needed. Her mind coalesced into a single cohesive personality. She ceased identifying as male and stopped taking cross-sex hormones. But by then, the damage was done.

She now suffers from a number of conditions related to taking testosterone: chronic hot flashes, genital pain, chronic joint pain, and suspected osteoporosis. She is suing the doctors who ignored her disabling psychological illnesses and instead treated her for the "gender dysphoria" that she didn't have, damaging her body in the process.

Is such a story unique? Unfortunately, no. If you'll recall, in an earlier chapter, Jamie Reed, a former case manager for a pediatric gender clinic, described how numerous severely mentally ill children, some with conditions like those Hannah/Layton suffered from, and some who didn't even want to "transition," were still given cross-sex hormones.

But there's one way in which her story might be different from those of others you've encountered in these pages. Layton's/Hannah's doctors practiced and treated her in Rhode Island. And even though years had passed before she realized how badly their "treatment" had hurt her, she might be able to get at least some recompense for what they did to her. That's because, although Rhode Island's statute of limitations for medical malpractice is just three years (meaning that a person injured by a doctor must sue within that time or is out of luck), Rhode Island expands the limits if the patient was disabled at the time of treatment due to mental incompetence.

Layton was in no condition to recognize that her doctors were hurting her at the time they were doing it. She was too incapacitated. Her doctors documented in her chart that she could barely function.

Medical malpractice statutes of limitations are typically just one to three years, depending on the state. In most cases where doctors cause a patient's injury, it's usually evident right away. But the vast majority of gender-confused people are mentally ill, often severely so. That makes them incapable of comprehending how dangerous these chemical and surgical body modifications and their side effects can be. When parents refuse to consent, gender doctors are ready with the drugs and scalpels the day these kids turn eighteen and can sign consent forms on their own. Gender specialists also have been accused, time and again, of inadequately explaining the effects and side effects, or of falsely claiming that the drugs like puberty blockers are fully reversible when they're not. So, a young person's future sexual function can be destroyed years before he or she even knows what sex is. And by the time he or she does, the doctor is legally off the hook.

Although a couple of dozen other detransitioners around the country have been able to sue, there might be tens of thousands more who would do so, if only the statute of limitations didn't bar them. Robert Weisenburger, of the California law firm LiMandri and Jonna, is among the attorneys working on three cases right now that allege injuries from chemical and surgical gender modifications. In all three cases, surgeons amputated the breasts of underage girls who once believed they were boys. The girls' ages were thirteen, fourteen, and fifteen, respectively, at the time of their surgeries. They all also were prescribed testosterone. Now young women, they've all been left with significant health conditions caused by such reckless medical and surgical interventions, as well as visible scars. Because they were minors when their "treatments" began, the California statute of limitations is three years instead of the usual one year in the state. Each was still under gender "treatment" within that three-year window before suing.

Weisenburger's firm has been contacted by numerous others who want to hold the doctors who "transitioned" them accountable. But the law firm has had to turn away most of them because of statute of limitations issues. Extending the time to sue would mean recourse for a great many more people.

"That's a very important way to protect these people's rights and to impose liability—create a significant liability exposure for medical professionals who are doing this," said Weisenburger. "Because without it, they're thoroughly protected from the harm that they're causing by these statutory limitations."

There are children, right now, who will never be able to experience orgasms as adults because their puberty was blocked when they were very young. Many of them will be sterile, as well. There is no way they could have consented to these losses at the age of eight, nine, ten, or eleven. And far more won't discover until years later how these brutal interventions predisposed them to the diseases that typically affect those much older, such as diabetes, heart disease, liver disease, osteoporosis, and reproductive system atrophy. They, too, are currently barred from seeking justice due to their states' statute of limitations on medical malpractice.

Even with just this handful of cases that were able to go forward, some insurers have responded by raising medical malpractice rates, or declining to cover trans procedures on minors. But that's not slowing down the trans train enough to make a difference.

Only when wantonly experimenting on children, the mentally ill, and otherwise vulnerable individuals becomes financially untenable will the medical/surgical aspect of the trans craze finally collapse.

The Executive Order Trump signed on January 28, 2025, titled "Protecting Children from Chemical and Surgical Mutilation," called for the Attorney General to work with Congress to "draft, propose, and promote legislation to enact a private right of action for children and the parents of children whose healthy body parts have been damaged by medical professionals practicing chemical and surgical mutilation, which should include a lengthy statute of limitations."

That's a good start. But I see two problems right away:

1. Such a statute almost certainly would not pass the Senate because it would be filibustered. It takes sixty votes to overcome the filibuster. There are one hundred senators. As of this writing, forty-seven of those senators are members of the Democratic Party. For some unfathomable reason, the party has chosen gender ideology as something it must defend at all costs. Would seven senators break ranks and vote aye? Doubtful.

2. Even if by some miracle such a bill does pass, it wouldn't protect all the young adults who fall victim to the ideology. The lack of parental consent hasn't stopped the clinics that already have kids lined up for surgery the moment they turn eighteen. A lengthy federal statute of limitations that protects only children under eighteen can't solve this problem.

What might? It's going to take a state-by-state effort.

Montana took the lead on this issue. Its state senate passed a bill that would have increased the statute of limitations for injuries caused by gender-related chemical and surgical malpractice. The bill sought to cover medical harms to both adults and children. Unfortunately, in the lower chamber, the bill was weakened, and the eventual law only covered minors. Had it also covered adults, it could have opened the floodgates.

I've heard through the grapevine that lawmakers in two other states have considered updating their relevant statutes. Could more state lawmakers, especially those who were at the forefront of prohibiting surgical and chemical gender procedures for minors, be persuaded to introduce similar laws?

Some of us might be able to play a role in ending these medical tragedies by bringing the medical statute of limitations problems to the attention of sympathetic state legislators. That's more likely to be successful if a state has previously passed laws to restrict puberty blockers, cross-sex hormones, or genital and breast removal surgeries for minors. But it's worth an attempt everywhere.

Open a dialogue with your state's lawmakers, either through social media or email, or by making an in-person appointment. Bring a copy of these pages with you. Explain that it typically takes many years before a person undergoing these procedures understands he or she has been irreparably injured.

Expand the statute of limitations in just a few states where legislators are amenable to protecting people from this madness, and the trickle of lawsuits we've seen so far will look like Niagara Falls.

And those currently profiting from the devastation will start looking into different specialties.

So, that's one idea to counter the transgender medical gravy train. But what about the schools where kids as young as five or six first learn from trusted teachers that they can swap sex just by saying so?

Teachers, administrators, and school board officials who promote transgenderism might be queer theory true believers, social justice warriors, virtue signalers, people who themselves identify outside of their sex, self-styled "glitter" substitutes for parents, or people just following the rules and trying to keep their jobs in a woke environment.

Parents around the country have sued schools, with varying degrees of success, under a variety of legal theories. The Fourteenth Amendment is often cited because the Supreme Court has found in the past that it protects the rights of parents to determine the upbringing of their children. But, win or lose, each case only affects those who bring it. Meanwhile, schools continue padding their curricula with trans propaganda while parents are kept in the dark.

What would force the ideology out of schools altogether? Could it be the First Amendment prohibition against the government establishing a religion? Because that's what some school systems are doing by promoting and sometimes mandating the teaching of gender ideology as fact. Transgenderism is a belief system. It's not based on anything real. You either accept it on faith or you don't.

Teaching children that they can change sex converts them to that belief system. Just as public school teachers would be trampling First Amendment prohibitions against the government establishing a religion if they were teaching kids to believe in the Koran, the Talmud, or Scientology's sacred scripture, they're overstepping those prohibitions by teaching children to believe in gender ideology. Yet, in many public schools today, more trans symbols, slogans, posters, and declarations are displayed in classrooms than there were symbols of Catholic belief in the Roman Catholic school of my youth.

Though this gender-based belief system doesn't require the worship of a deity, not all religions do. Buddhism, Taoism, Jainism, and Scientology are religions that also don't involve worshipping a particular god or gods. With or without deities, no one questions that these are religions. And if anyone did try to preach Scientology's sacred scripture in a public school, they'd be shut down pretty quickly. So why do we tolerate teachers preaching transgenderism?

I'd ask any lawyers reading right now to consider whether we can get trans ideology out of schools the same way that previous generations fought and won against schools that merely displayed the Ten Commandments.

Two cases currently winding their way through the federal court system at least partly base their complaints on First Amendment grounds. In one case, teachers in Escondido, California, objected on religious grounds to being coerced into lying to parents when their kids adopted new "identities" at school. The deception went against the teachers' faith. The judge in that case, quoting an older case, denied the school system's request to dismiss the complaint And the quote he chose shows that he understood this to be a profound assault on First Amendment rights not to be converted to a new religion by a public school:

*Families entrust public schools with the education of their children, but condition their trust on the understanding that the classroom will not purposely be **used to advance religious views** that may conflict with the private beliefs of the student and his or her family.* [emphasis added]

In other words, public school officials do not have the right to proselytize other people's kids to their faith.

The second case that puts the First Amendment front and center comes from the other side of the struggle, the side that wants free rein to socially, chemically, and surgically transform children into facsimiles of the opposite sex.

PFLAG is a nonprofit that promotes gender ideology. Represented by lawyers with the ACLU and LAMBDA, it filed a federal lawsuit opposing Trump's Executive Orders "Protecting Children from Chemical and Surgical Mutilation" and "Defending Women from Gender Ideology Extremism and Restoring Biological Truth to the Federal Government." The lawsuit claimed that these Executive Orders discriminated against people who reject their birth sex by withholding federal funding for trans-related activities and body modifications and the promotion of gender ideology.

One of the bases for PFLAG's complaint is this:

By withholding federal grants, the Orders engage in unconstitutional viewpoint discrimination in violation of the First Amendment and violate the rights of grant recipients and transgender patients.

Attorney Kara Dansky found that argument "astonishing" and highlighted it in her online newsletter, *The Terf Report*:

*. . . if it is a belief system, or a mere viewpoint (**which we have been saying this entire time**), then it cannot be innate and **there should literally be no need for anyone to go on puberty blockers and/or opposite-sex hormones to 'affirm' it**.* [emphasis in the original]

This will be a long fight and those of us who see the risks to our families and to society as a whole need our own alliances to combat the forces on the other side. Whether you realize it or not, there are probably people all around you right now who agree that this is wrong but aren't necessarily speaking up. In a 2022 poll, 70 percent of respondents said they were against teaching gender identity in schools. Others you know are likely to be persuadable, if only they knew all that you do after reading this book.

One way to become active in your local community is to find out whether there's a Moms for Liberty chapter in your area. While Moms for Liberty started as a conservative group, and many chapters are still overwhelmingly conservative, plenty of liberals and moderates who are concerned about transgenderism being introduced in public schools have also become involved.

As Carter's mom Ellie spoke about in an earlier chapter, liberals have been primed by their preferred news and entertainment media to see conservatives as knuckle-draggers who are wrong about everything. But conservatives were right about gender ideology. Most know more about how vulnerable children and young adults with mental health problems are being indoctrinated into the trans cult than the average liberal or moderate does.

The irony here is that it's the liberal and moderate families whose kids are most at risk, because of laws in the places where most of us live and the policies of our liberal and progressive school districts.

It doesn't matter where we fall on the political spectrum. We have more in common with our fellow citizens than not, despite how our political and media personalities try to divide us. We have to work together to protect our kids and our society.

Some of us have already been reaching out to the "other side." We don't agree on everything, but we don't have to. On this one issue, we are united: safeguard the young.

Others you've met in the pages of this book come from the liberal end of the political spectrum, including Erin Friday, Jeannette Cooper, Beth Bourne, Stephanie Winn, Grace Ellison, Kim Jones, Alesha Perkins, and several more. That hasn't stopped them from working hand-in-hand with conservatives to end medical and surgical experimentation on kids; to end indoctrination, sexualization, and social transitioning in schools; and to fight to retain the rights of parents, as well as those of women and girls.

Beyond the battle against those who promote transgenderism, we have to examine the ways we ourselves might have unwittingly helped the ideology to thrive.

Some of us have dutifully called anyone who identifies out of their sex by pronouns that don't match their sex. Even some journalists who write about how dangerous the ideology is to kids nevertheless regularly use female pronouns when referring to male AGPs and transvestic fetishists.

I understand that people want to be kind, or polite. As I pointed out in the Introduction, I've been there. But here's the funny thing about language: it shapes our sense of reality. Call a man a woman (or vice versa) and pretty soon, you'll start seeing that man as a woman.

We have to retrain ourselves to use the language correctly, as we learned to do when growing up. Call men what they are: men. It's a three-letter word. It's not an insult. And women, even those with facial hair and receding hairlines due to injecting testosterone, are still women. They always will be. Retrain yourself to see them and refer to them as they are.

If you find yourself slightly panicked at the idea of using accurate language to refer to someone's sex, you're experiencing the power of manipulation. You've been coerced into pretending this belief system is real. Maybe you fear the repercussions that come with acknowledging what you know to be true.

But why are we hiding from the truth?

If we want change, the first thing we have to change is that emotional reaction that warns us against subscribing to truth and accuracy.

Gender means sex. Activists might argue that sex and gender mean separate things. But those same activists also demand that everyone claiming a different "gender" be treated as if that person were the opposite sex.

So, again, gender is sex. People born with penises are male. People capable of giving birth are female. These are facts that don't change. If we use language in a way meant to obscure these facts, we contribute to the trans craze.

Whenever we refer to a man as "she," we concede ground on biological reality. We help to obscure the fact that no man belongs in a room where little girls undress. And we make it that much more difficult to keep the next man who claims a trans identity from exposing himself to those girls because we've played along with the fantasy that he, too, is some version of a "girl."

Surrender on the language and you've granted him a license. Train yourself to stop. Now.

I won't claim that it will be easy. Unreality has replaced reality in so many situations, and many of us have gone along and now barely notice. I have close friends whose son has gone through all the body modification surgeries that help him mimic a woman, and who takes cross-sex hormones. They call him their daughter. Although they already know my position on transgenderism, this book might end my friendship with them and with others who believe that getting real about which sex is which is bigotry.

If that happens, I will regret the losses, but if we don't steel ourselves to tolerate possible rejection, and perhaps worse, from those we like, and perhaps even some we love, we won't be able to get to the other side of this.

So accept that you're going to be labeled and that there are those who will try to discredit you in other ways.

Is standing up for the truth worth all that?

Look at what's happened so far while most of us slept through the takeover. Can tolerating the discomfort that might result from acknowledging reality be any worse?

Aside from the immediate need to protect children and young adults, we also have to consider what kind of society we want to live in going forward. And, again, the risk goes beyond transgenderism to all the ways that queer theorists want to "queer" anything that could get in the way of normalizing all manner of sexual behavior.

Even some psychology professionals who are skeptical of gender claims have been urging the destigmatization of so-called virtuous pedophiles (those who, presumably, don't act on their attractions).

This is the next battlefront. Pedophiles (or "minor-attracted persons," as some call themselves), have been trying to attach themselves to the alphabet soup of LGBTQIAA++ for years. If society doesn't defend its norms and values as essential to a healthy culture, eventually, they *will* succeed.

Look what happened when we destigmatized tranvestic fetishism/autogynephilia. That, on the surface, seemed relatively victimless, but the fetishists now demand to be treated in every respect as women.

We're a tolerant society. But with unlimited tolerance, nothing on queer theory's wish list can be kept in check.

Don't be cowed by labels or smears. Forge new alliances to counter the one that's foisted this madness on us.

Unqueer the queering. Disrupt the disruption. And let's get back to reality.

Acknowledgments

Writing might be a solitary profession, yet no writer of nonfiction will accomplish much without the help of others.

She alone might analyze the information she uncovers, arrange it in logical sequence on the page, decide how to phrase her points so that their meanings are easily grasped by her eventual readers. But the sources of all that she uncovers, analyzes, and phrases? There are likely to be thousands of them, including countless individuals who confide their stories, provide expert insights on arcane issues, help her make connections to others with relevant information, and supply pertinent documents.

How can I ever thank all those who helped make this book possible? That, in itself, might take an entire book. But a few people stand out and deserve mention.

Let me start by expressing my gratitude to my friend and colleague Chris Adamec, a talented health and science writer, who reviewed every chapter as I wrote it. I persevered in large part thanks to her encouragement and keen eye.

I also owe thanks to my son, Alex Tomaino, who patiently listened as I poured out my distress each time I learned of a new horror being inflicted on a young person or her family. Having Alex as a sounding board helped me decompress.

Many thanks, too, to therapist Stephanie Winn, host of the podcast *You Must Be Some Kind of Therapist*, associate producer of the documentary on detransitioners, *No Way Back*, and champion of parents of gender-confused children. Stephanie became my go-to expert on the psychological damage inflicted on the young and vulnerable by gender ideologues. She also introduced me to several people who were currently attempting, or had previously attempted, to mimic the opposite sex. And she put me in touch with a number of medical and mental health professionals who have been on the front lines of the gender wars.

And I can never thank Ellie Keenan enough for connecting me with so many people whose lives were turned upside down due to gender madness. Though we might be on opposite sides on many other issues, we seemed to be of one mind when it came to protecting the vulnerable from gender ideology.

Immense appreciation goes out to all the parents, teens, young adults, mental health professionals, doctors, lawyers, and others who trusted me with their stories and insights. Although not every interviewee was quoted in the final draft, what you shared helped me better understand this mass psychogenic illness, and how it spread. So, even if I haven't specifically named you in the text, please know that your contributions are in here and were indispensable.

A few parents in particular deserve special mention: Alesha Perkins, Beth Bourne, Erin Friday, Erin Lee, and Jeanette Cooper. Each of these moms has become a crusader, determined to do what she can to help other parents counter the seductive power of the trans cult.

Lastly, a special thank you to Kurt Volkan, publisher of Pitchstone Publishing, who helped me refine and narrow the scope of the work. Kurt had the courage to publish *Sacrificial Lambs* along with several other books that document the damage done by gender ideology while much of the rest of the book publishing world was serving up empty-headed tomes promoting it.

This book is dedicated to all of you.

Appendix I: The Effects and Limits of Trump's Executive Orders

I spent some time speaking with attorney and author Kara Dansky—a lifelong leftist Democrat who is a past president of Women's Declaration International USA—to better understand the effects and limits of President Donald Trump's Executive Orders on gender, in particular the one titled "Defending Women from Gender Ideology Extremism and Restoring Biological Truth to the Federal Government."

What does such an Executive Order (EO) give the government the power to do?

"The language [of the EO] is, 'Agencies shall take all necessary steps as permitted by law to end the federal funding of gender ideology,'" said Dansky. "Virtually every United States educational institution receives funding under Title IX, which prohibits sex discrimination in education. And so depending on how all this plays out, it's possible that if schools refuse to comply with this order, then the Department of Education could remove their federal funding."

As Dansky explained, the authority to cut funding if schools don't comply doesn't come from the EO itself, but from existing law. That law is Title IX. It had been reinterpreted by the previous administration to prohibit discrimination, not on the basis of sex, but on the basis of gender identity. The previous administration then promulgated regulations to enforce its new interpretation, which prohibited discrimination on the basis of "gender identity." As a result, under President Joe Biden, Title IX's ability to prevent discrimination on the basis of sex was obviated.

Any boy who claimed to have a girl's "gender identity" had to be accommodated as if female were his actual sex. Wherever that happened, girls lost their rights to privacy in bathrooms, locker rooms, and elsewhere. And they lost their rights to fair play in sports any time boys wanted to play on their teams.

Several states sued over the Biden administration's Title IX changes. Just days prior to Biden leaving office, a federal court found that his administration's changes violated the Constitution, exceeded the administration's authority, and were arbitrary and capricious. The presiding judge wrote that:

> *Put simply, there is nothing in the text or statutory design of Title IX to suggest that discrimination "on the basis of sex" means anything other than it has since Title IX's inception—that recipients of federal funds under Title IX may not treat a person worse than another similarly-situated individual on the basis of the person's sex, i.e., male or female.*

So, discrimination on the basis of gender identity is no longer a Title IX issue; it has reverted to its original meaning. The current administration can enforce the law as intended: to protect females from discrimination on the basis of sex. And the Trump administration (and subsequent administrations) can write regulations that detail how the government should do that.

But Trump's EO goes further. It includes sections that define the two sexes:

Sec. 3. Recognizing Women Are Biologically Distinct From Men.

(a) Within 30 days of the date of this order, the Secretary of Health and Human Services shall provide to the U.S. Government, external partners, and the public clear guidance expanding on the sex-based definitions set forth in this order.

(b) Each agency and all Federal employees shall enforce laws governing sex-based rights, protections, opportunities, and accommodations to protect men and women as biologically distinct sexes. Each agency should therefore give the terms "sex", "male", "female", "men", "wom-

en", "boys" and "girls" the meanings set forth in section 2 of this order when interpreting or applying statutes, regulations, or guidance and in all other official agency business, documents, and communications.

(c) When administering or enforcing sex-based distinctions, every agency and all Federal employees acting in an official capacity on behalf of their agency shall use the term "sex" and not "gender" in all applicable Federal policies and documents . . .

*Sec. 6. Bill Text. Within 30 days of the date of this order, **the Assistant to the President for Legislative Affairs shall present to the President proposed bill text to codify the definitions in this order**.* [emphasis added]

The section on "Bill Text" is worth noting. To "codify" the definitions means to write a federal law that affirms that there are only two sexes, male and female, and that gender identity " . . . does not provide a meaningful basis for identification and cannot be recognized as a replacement for sex."

Congress would have to pass such law. If it does, rules that enforce gender identity would be more difficult to resurrect in subsequent administrations.

Bizarre as this seems, there's no guarantee that a law that simply acknowledges there are only two sexes would pass. Democrats, though in the minority, could block it in the Senate.

"I do know that a vast majority of Americans across the political spectrum understand that there only two sexes and that sex is immutable," said Dansky.

True, but politicians are interested in keeping their jobs. And in "blue" states, voters could penalize a senator for voting for any law that states the obvious. There are only male and female. Sperm and egg. There are no additional sexes or gametes. One can't change into the other, no matter how fervently a person might wish it to be so.

It's also not certain that progressive cities and states will comply with any regulations that the current administration writes to stop their public schools from teaching gender ideology, that assure privacy and fair play for girls, or that prohibit schools from "socially transitioning" children without permission or notice to children's parents.

This opinion comes from a second attorney, Candice Jackson. Jackson had helped write Title IX regulations in the first Trump administration and is currently the Deputy General Counsel for the US Department of Education, where she authored the Trump EO, "Keeping Men Out of Women's Sports."

In a webinar, Jackson explained that states could tell school districts to turn down the federal money they would forfeit by choosing to continue their gender policies, with the state making up the difference. That's possible because the federal government provides only about 10 percent of K–12 public school budgets, on average. And it appears to be what some states are considering as I write this.

Jackson believes that the effects will be greater at colleges and universities. The reason for this? Almost all colleges are subject to Title IX and other federal regulations because they let their students apply for federal financial aid. And in higher education, that federal money can make up a significant portion of the schools' funding.

Chase Strangio of the ACLU and Shannon Minter of the National Center for Lesbian Rights, both lawyers, and both women who identify as men, have indicated that their organizations and others that support and promote gender ideology are busily filing and preparing to file legal challenges against implementation of several of the gender-related Executive Orders.

As I write this, legal challenges have already been filed against the EO titled "Protecting Children from Chemical and Surgical Mutilation," which prohibits federal funds from being used to provide drugs and surgeries to those under the age of nineteen. Because the EO is not a law, it can't stop doctors and hospitals from continuing to damage the healthy bodies of young people. But it does order the federal government to stop funding institutions that perform those procedures on young people. Unless a court overrules the EO, at minimum, doctors and hospitals won't be able to bill Medicare, Medicaid, and Tricare to pay for puberty blockers, cross-sex hormones, or surgical interventions meant to make a body resemble that of the opposite sex.

The "Defending Women from Gender Ideology Extremism ... " EO that recognizes there are only two sexes also orders that male federal prisoners be removed from federal prisons for women. (This EO has no effect on state-run facilities where the vast majority of prisoners are housed.) As of this writing, several male federal prisoners who were scheduled to be transferred to male facilities have filed a lawsuit and had their transfers put on hold.

That EO might also affect how the Equal Employment Opportunity Commission (EEOC) prioritizes complaints of workplace discrimination. During the Biden administration, a man who identified as a woman probably would have found the EEOC eager to back up his demands to use woman's bathrooms, showers, changing rooms, and other female-only facilities at his workplace. Under the current EO, that same agency is more likely to defend the rights of women to single-sex spaces, and to investigate claims of workplace harassment and discrimination if women complain of being forced to share intimate facilities with males.

Appendix II: Advice to Parents

Among the most damaging changes we've seen from trans madness are the assaults on the rights of parents to keep their families whole and to protect their children.

Below, you'll find some documents written by others that can help parents understand and navigate this strange new landscape.

If you're a parent, even if you don't believe your kids have been exposed to indoctrination, it pays to be vigilant. No parent I interviewed for this book thought his or her child was at risk—not one—until after the child adopted a trans persona.

Don't wait for the evidence that transgenderism has snuck in through the basement window. Block it at the front door.

If you have friends who are parents, share these resources with them.

The first step is to be informed. And a good place to start gathering information is at your child's school. Erin Friday, a California mom and attorney who almost lost her daughter to the trans cult, and the co-lead of the US chapter of Our Duty, created the following document that parents can send to schools to request their kids' records. Making such requests isn't foolproof. Some schools have gone to elaborate lengths to hide evidence that a child has adopted a wrong-sex identity. But it's a start. Federal law is on your side, even though not every school will comply, and there might also be laws in the state where you live that protect your rights. When you're fighting for the right to parent your own children against those who believe they know better than you, persistence is essential.

Advice for Requesting Information from Schools

Send this request every month to see if your school is transitioning your child behind your back. You never know when the school will finally trick your child into believing that he or she was born wrong and must adopt a gender identity in order to be authentic.

Dear Superintendent [ ] and Principal [ ]:

This letter is to request access to records in the possession of the _____ School District and _____ School, including all members of school boards, superintendents, school counselors, teachers and staff (collectively, the "Schools"), for the purpose of inspection and copying pursuant to the Family Educational Rights and Privacy Act (FERPA).

I am the parent of [child's legal name]. The information that I ask to inspect is as follows:

1. For the time period of [dates that cover the entire period your child has attended the school], all records, documents, reports, memoranda, writings, notes, emails, text messages, and any electronic records of [child's legal name] born on [child's birth date] (the "Pupil") inclusive of official and unofficial, "shadow files" and social transition plans, or records evidencing that the School is using a different name for the Pupil than his/her legal name.

2. For the time period of [dates that cover the entire period your child has attended the school], all records, documents, reports, memoranda, writings, notes, emails, text messages, and any electronic records related, referring to, or discussing the name and pronoun that is to be used when communicating with Pupil at _____ School (including teachers, administration, and staff.)

3. For the time period of [dates that cover the entire period your child has attended the school], all records, documents, reports, memoranda, writings, notes, emails, text messages, and any electronic records related, referring to, or discussing the Pupil's gender identity.

4. For the time period of [dates that cover the entire period your child has attended the school], all records, documents, reports, memoranda, writings, notes, emails, text messages, and any electronic records related, referring to, or discussing the Pupil's parents.

5. For the time period [dates that cover the entire period your child has attended the school], all records, documents, reports, memoranda, notes, emails, text messages, and any electronic records related, referring to, or discussing whether to keep the Pupil's chosen name and pronoun confidential from Pupil's parents.

6. For the time period of [dates that cover the entire period your child has attended the school], all of Pupil's records, reports, memoranda, writings, emails, text messages, and other electronic records maintained by any third party.

7. For the time period of [dates that cover the entire period your child has attended the school], all of Pupil's records, reports, memoranda, writings, emails, text messages, and other electronic records maintained by any third party of Pupil's social media kept or tracked by _____ School or any third party.

8. For the time periods [dates that cover the entire period your child has attended the school], all emails between my child and each of her/his teachers [name the teachers].

This request reasonably describes identifiable records or information to be produced from that record.

Request for Information in Electronic Format

I am seeking these records in any and all electronic formats your office keeps them in. **My request extends to receipt of this information in any and all electronic formats your office maintains these records in, except emails should be in pdf format.** Delivery of this information to me by electronic mail [insert your email address here] or via a thumb drive or via a disk is fine. I can supply the District with a thumb drive if needed. *Please advise what electronic format these records are kept in.*

In addition, if there are documents that satisfy this request that are in **both** electronic and paper formats, *please provide the electronic version of those records*. It is hoped that this will save the District and me time, trouble, and expense.

If you anticipate that data compilation, extraction, or programming will be required to satisfy a request, please provide a written estimate and justification for same. Given the high profile of this matter with the public and the recentness of the date of any responsive records, a compilation, extraction, or programming should not be required to obtain responsive documents.

I ask that you make the record(s) promptly available, for inspection and copying, based on my payment of fees covering direct costs of duplication, or statutory fee, if applicable.

If any portion of the information I have requested is exempt from discovery, express provisions of law require segregation and deletion of that material in order that the remainder of the information may be released. If you determine that an express provision of law exists to exempt disclosure of all or a portion of the material I have requested, provide me with notification as to the reasons for the determination not later than 10 days from your receipt of this request.

Thank you for your prompt attention to my request.

Respectfully,

SIGNATURE

NAME

(Source: Erin Friday, OurDuty.group)

Advice for Overseeing Your Child's Online Access

If you know or suspect that your child has been exposed to trans propaganda at school, online, or elsewhere, it's vital to counteract those influences.

A mother who wants to be identified only as "Fed Up Colorado Mom" shared her strategies on the website Parents With Inconvenient Truths About Trans. Monitoring and controlling what her daughter was able to access online, and who she was able to interact with, eventually helped her teen daughter desist from a trans identity.

The Bark phone this mom mentions was a key part of her strategy. It's designed to allow parents to control what websites kids can visit and who can contact them. Several other companies also offer phones with parental controls, but as of this writing, Bark appears to be have more features and be the most customizable.

Spoiler alert: kids hate these phones. The daughter of "Fed Up" raged for weeks when her mom took away her iPhone and gave her the Bark in its place. And "Fed Up" says that monitoring is a full-time job in itself, something I've heard from other parents who've ordered parental-control phones for their teens. But when you consider the alternative, annoying your child with a limited function phone seems worth it. Here's "Fed Up's" account:

> We heavily restricted internet in the beginning. We showed her articles and watched a few videos on how social media is horrible for children and let her know we would not be doing our jobs as parents if we didn't take this seriously and that we had made a mistake by allowing unlimited access in the past. I even went so far as to lock all the Netflix profiles with an age restriction and manually removed titles from what was available for my kids (Heartstopper, for example).
>
> You can do this from your online parent account. Just Google what shows have "trans" or "LGBTQ" themes on Netflix and block it from their profile.
>
> My daughter was never too heavily into anime, but liked Kipo and She-Ra and Nimona. I let her have Netflix back after I cleaned it up. We still don't allow YouTube on her personal phone or laptop, but she watches it at school.
>
> We slowly gave her Instagram back after about six months but only with the contingency that she allow me to supervise it and log in as her at any time. I am logged in as her on my phone and so get all her notifications, etc.
>
> I have still blocked any roleplay sites (like Warrior Cats). She did return to playing some Roblox with friends she's known forever and does have access to Discord to call her friends while she's playing

it. Same thing, I am logged in as her on Discord so have full access to everything.

The Bark phone also still monitors everything so, if she is using an alt account, I would still be notified of inappropriate chats/content, etc. She is still time restricted online.

We focus on getting out of the house first, doing chores, playing games, etc., before we get online. I want it to be a last resort. It is hard because she likes drawing and loves trading drawings with the online art community, but of course, almost every character people send to her to draw has "top surgery" scars on them, or is LGBTQ or trans.

After a while it really gets to my daughter. She now sees how this stuff is everywhere. I think most parents have NO CLUE how crazy rampant this stuff is online and what their kids are being exposed to, especially if they're into the art or fantasy stuff online. They grow up thinking all of this is normal and that it's no big deal being trans or having your breasts surgically removed. It's really screwing up a lot of our kids along with all of the adults promoting this stuff. It's a travesty.

(Source: pittparents.com)

Advice for Reaching Your Trans-Identified Child

Therapist Stephanie Winn, who hosts a popular podcast that focuses on the trans craze, also offers an online course and a community forum for parents whose kids have adopted trans identities. Many parents are stumped about how to respond when their children get indoctrinated into the trans cult. The following, excerpted with permission from her course, "ROGD Repair," provides some advice about how to reach your kid when your kid isn't willing to listen:

Many parents find themselves in gridlock when they attempt to persuade their child by insisting that they consider written or other educational material, such as books, peer-reviewed journal articles, or detransitioner stories. As I've expressed elsewhere in this course, pushing your child too hard can backfire, ultimately rendering them more rigid and less able to hear your valid concerns.

Other parents may default in the opposite direction, overly concealing their knowledge and opinions for fear it will spark massive conflict. Yet this strategy alone, when left to fester, may mean that your child never gets exposed to the truth about what "gender transition" really entails, and how it affects people.

Leaving reading material lying around is an alternative, middle path that may be more compatible with adolescents' self-consciousness, rebelliousness, need for privacy, and resistance to authority. They can pick it up and put it down at will, when you aren't looking, never giving you the satisfaction of knowing that they looked, or hearing what they thought.

Should they challenge you on it in an inappropriate manner, such as yelling or calling you names ("bigot," "transphobe"), you have every right to set appropriate boundaries about how you will be treated, and remind them that in your home, you get to read whatever you want.

(Source: ROGDrepair.com)

Resources

Numerous organizations offer information and support for anyone who has been harmed by the gender industry or who wants to know more about what the research actually says about gender confusion and the effects of gender ideology, and a number of podcasts regularly or often discuss the topics and themes covered in this book.

Organizations

Democrats for an Informed Approach to Gender (www.di-ag.org): An online gathering place for liberals who have been affected by gender ideology. Visit this site to find information, swap stories with others, and learn about how and where to take action.

Detrans Help (detranshelp.org): A nonprofit run by detransitioners for detransitioners, dedicated to helping those who were once seduced by gender ideology.

4th Wave Now (4thwavenow.com): Posts stories and information about transgenderism, news about research, and commentaries.

Genspect (genspect.org): Genspect advocates for a non-medical approach to gender distress and hosts a number of online and in-person events to provide information and support to those affected by gender ideology and those who want to know more. Genspect also has a page that ranks colleges according to their degree of trans activism: college.genspect.org.

Our Duty (ourduty.group): This international group advocates for keeping children safe from gender ideology and connects parents to each other for support.

Parents With Inconvenient Truths About Trans (pittparents.com): A site for parents of teens and young adults who've lost their kids to the trans craze to tell their personal stories and to give and get support. A number of these parents have also shared the welcome news that their children have since desisted from believing they are a different sex.

Parents of ROGD Kids (parentsofrogdkids.com/support-groups): Connects parents with local support groups.

Society for Evidence-Based Gender Medicine (segm.org): This site was founded by medical professionals and researchers and posts accurate information about medical research into gender issues.

The Terf Report (karadansky.substack.com): Attorney Kara Dansky helps readers understand the legal and political ramifications of actions by those who promote the ideology and those who oppose it.

Themis Resource Fund (themisresourcefund.org): A nonprofit organization that connects detransitioners in the United States with attorneys. It also assists with funds for litigation.

Podcasts

Gender: A Wider Lens, produced by Genspect (genspect.org/resources/gender-a-wider-lens/)

You Must Be Some Kind of Therapist with Stephanie Winn (sometherapist.com)

Calmversations with Benjamin Boyce (youtube.com/c/benjaminaboyce)

Andrew Gold, Heretics (youtube.com/@andrewgoldheretics)

The Megyn Kelly Show (megynkelly.com)

Notes

Introduction

8   *Children taught they are either oppressed or oppressors:* Charlie Peters, "No, We Don't Need to 'Decolonise' Nurseries," *Spiked Online,* May 12, 2022, www.spiked-online.com/2022/05/12/no-we-dont-need-to-decolonise-nurseries/. *See also*: Paulo Freire, *Pedagogy of the Oppressed* (Bloomsbury Academic, 2018).

9   *Queer theory intertwines deviant sex with social justice issues:* Gayle S. Rubin, "Thinking Sex: Notes for a Radical Theory of the Politics of Sexuality," in *Pleasure and Danger: Exploring Female Sexuality*, ed. Carol S. Vance (Routledge & Kegan Paul 1984), 143–179.

Alec Shemmel, "1st Grade Teachers Tells Students Doctors 'Make a Guess about Gender When Baby Is Born," *KOMO News,* April, 11, 2022, komonews.com/news/nation-world/1st-grade-teacher-tells-students-doctors-make-a-guess-about-gender-when-a-baby-is-born-boston-massachusetts-ray-skyer-transgender.

Queer theory inspired sex ed: Advocates for Youth, *Rights, Respect, Responsibility: A K–12 Sex Education Curriculum*, www.advocatesforyouth.org/resources/rights-respect-responsibility-a-k-12-sex-education-curriculum/.

Teaching kids they can avoid the "wrong" puberty: Planned Parenthood's Teen Council (Washington state), "Puberty," 18–19 (last updated February 2020).

Black Lives Matter at School's thirteen "Guiding Principles" for schools: Black Lives Matter at School, "Guiding Principles," www.blacklivesmatteratschool.com/guiding-principles.html.

10   Dr. Marci Bowers, in an interview by Margaret Brennan, *Face the Na-*

246

tion, July 23, 2023, www.cbsnews.com/news/marci-bowers-world-professional-association-for-transgender-health-president-face-the-nation-transcript-07-23-2023/.

Estimates of minors getting gender surgeries: Jason D. Wright, MD, et al., "National Estimates of Gender-Affirming Surgery in the US," *JAMA Network Open*, August 23, 2023, doi:10.1001/jamanetworkopen.2023.30348.

11   *Dr. Marci Bowers surgically inverts 17-year-old Jazz Jennings' penis*: "It's a Girl!" *I Am Jazz*, season 5, episode 5 (TLC, January 29, 2019), www.tlc.com/shows/i-am-jazz/episodes/its-a-girl.

12   *2013 DSM-5 estimates of all those who met the diagnostic criteria for gender dysphoria*: *The Diagnostic and Statistical Manual of Mental Disorders*, 5th ed. (DSM–5) (American Psychiatric Association, 2013), 451–460.

13   *Williams Institute 2017 estimates, 13- to 17-year-olds who believed themselves to be transgender:* Jody L. Herman et al. "Age of Individuals Who Identify as Transgender in the United States," Williams Institute, UCLA School of Law, January 2017, 2, williamsinstitute.law.ucla.edu/wp-content/uploads/Age-Trans-Individuals-Jan-2017.pdfuj8bcv.

Williams Institute 2022 estimates, 13- to 17-year-olds who believed themselves to be transgender: Jody L. Herman et al., "How Many Adults and Youth Identify as Transgender in the United States?," Williams Institute, UCLA School of Law, January 2022, 1, williamsinstitute.law.ucla.edu/wp-content/uploads/Trans-Pop-Update-Jun-2022.pdf.

CDC survey finds 5.5% of high schoolers say they're trans or think they might be: Nicolas A. Suarez, MPH, et al., "Disparities in School Connectedness, Unstable Housing, Experiences of Violence, Mental Health, and Suicidal Thoughts and Behaviors Among Transgender and Cisgender High School Students—Youth Risk Behavior Survey," MMWR Supplement (US Department of Health and Human Services, Centers for Disease Control and Prevention, October 10, 2024).

14   *Referrals to UK gender clinic increase dramatically:* Gordon Rayner, "Minister Orders Inquiry into 4,000% Rise in Children Wanting to Change Sex," *Telegraph*, September 16, 2018, www.telegraph.co.uk/politics/2018/09/16/minister-orders-inquiry-4000-per-cent-rise-children-wanting/.

Cross-dressing paraphilias in straight males can begin in adolescence: Zucker et al., "Demographics, Behavior Problems, and Psychosexual Characteristics of Adolescents with Gender Identity Disorder or Transvestic Fetishism," *Journal of Sex & Marital Therapy*, March 5 2012, doi.org/10.1080/0092623X.2011.611219.

Adolescent-onset gender dysphoria in girls is a new phenomenon: Lisa Littman, "Parent Reports of Adolescents and Young Adults Perceived to Show Signs of a Rapid Onset of Gender Dysphoria," *PLOS One,* August 16, 2018, doi.org/10.1371/journal.pone.0202330; Karl Bradford Jones, MD, FAAFP, "Mass Psychogenic Illness," *Family Doctor,* familydoctor.org/condition/mass-psychogenic-illness/ (last updated January 2024).

15   *Gender dysphoria typically resolves in adolescence rather than suddenly appearing then:* Littman, "Parent Reports of Adolescents and Young Adults."

Second-grade sex ed curriculum includes vocabulary memorization words "vulva," "scrotum," and "clitoris," but "boy" and "girl" are missing, referred to only by their genitals: Unit 3: Growth and Development + Violence Prevention, 2nd Grade, Portland, Oregon, acquired via public records request.

Explicit images of genitalia in fourth- and fifth-grade sex ed lessons: Planned Parenthood's Teen Council (Washington state), "Puberty," 18–19. See also: "External Anatomy – Body with a Vulva," 5th Grade, Unit 3: Growth and Development + Violence Prevention, Portland, Oregon, acquired via public records request.

17   James Bickerton, "Misgendering Should Be a Crime, According to Millennials," *Newsweek,* July 15, 2023, www.newsweek.com/misgendering-should-crime-according-millennials-1813178.

People threatened with or actually imprisoned in other countries for "misgendering": See succeeding chapters.

18   *About 75% of men claiming to be women are acting out an extreme fetish-like paraphilia:* J. Michael Bailey, PhD, and Ray Blanchard, PhD, "Gender Dysphoria Is Not One Thing," 4th Wave Now, December 7, 2017, 4thwavenow.com/2017/12/07/gender-dysphoria-is-not-one-thing/.

Experts with differing views on who is a transvestic fetishist and who is an AGP: Dr. Az Hakeem, "Frauds, Fetishes, and Frameworks in Today's Trans Movement," *Gender: A Wider Lens,* interview by Stella O'Malley and Sasha Ayed, November 15, 2024, www.youtube.com/watch?v=aHe5vbMj_YU, versus George R. Brown, MD, "Transvestic Disorder," *Merck Manual,* Professional Edition, revised 2023.

19   *Males overtaking female sports:* "Report of the Special Rapporteur on Violence Against Women and Girls, Its Causes and Consequences," United Nations 79th Session, Item 27 of the Provisional Agenda, Advancement of Women, August 27, 2024, docs.un.org/en/A/79/325.

Almost half of male federal prisoners who claim to be trans are sex offenders: May Mailman et al., "Cruel and Unusual Punishment," Independent Women's Forum 2024, 20.

Chapter One: The Myth of the Magical Child

23 *After the rest of the body is grown, the brain is still immature:* "The Teen Brain: Seven Things to Know," National Institute of Mental Health, revised 2023, www.nimh.nih.gov/health/publications/the-teen-brain-7-things-to-know.

24 Ed Yong, "Young Trans Children Know Who They Are," *Atlantic,* January 15, 2019, www.theatlantic.com/science/archive/2019/01/young-trans-children-know-who-they-are/580366/.

25 *Almost all desist from gender distress by adulthood:* Alex Byrne, "Another Myth of Persistence?," *Archives of Sexual Behavior,* June 17, 2024, doi.org/10.1007/s10508-024-03005-1; Kristina Olson et al., "Mental Health of Transgender Children Who Are Supported in Their Identities," *Pediatrics,* March 1, 2016, doi.org/10.1542/peds.2015-3223.
Zucker on social transitioning of children leading to persistence: K. Zucker, "Debate: Different Strokes for Different Folks," *Child and Adolescent Mental Health,* May 31, 2019, doi:10.1111/camh.12330.

26 *I Am Jazz* (TLC), www.tlc.com/shows/i-am-jazz.

27 *Jazz Jennings' surgery complications:* Aurellie Corinthios, "Jazz Jennings' Doctors Say She Had a 'Difficult Surgical Course' with a 'Severe' Complication," *People,* January 22, 2020, people.com/tv/jazz-jennings-doctors-say-she-had-a-difficult-surgical-course-with-a-severe-complication/.
Olson wins MacArthur Genius Award: "Kristina Olson, psychologist, Class of 2018: Advancing the scientific understanding of gender and shedding light on the social and cognitive development of transgender and gender-nonconforming youth," MacArthur Foundation, www.macfound.org/fellows/class-of-2018/kristina-olson.
Kristina Olson et al., "Mental Health of Transgender Children Who Are Supported in Their Identities," *Pediatrics,* March 1, 2016, doi.org/10.1542/peds.2015-3223.
Zucker fired: Jesse Singal, "How the Fight Over Transgender Kids Got a Leading Sex Researcher Fired," *Cut,* February 7, 2016, www.thecut.com/2016/02/fight-over-trans-kids-got-a-researcher-fired.html.
Gender confusion is rarely lifelong: Alex Byrne, "Another Myth of Per-

sistence?" *Archives of Sexual Behavior*, June 17, 2024, doi.org/10.1007/s10508-024-03005-1.

29   *Function of GnRH:* Arjang Naim, MD, "Gonadotropin Releasing Hormone (GnRH),"drarjangnaim.com/gonadotropin-releasing-hormone-gnrh/.

Negative effects of puberty blockers on children: Tingley vs. Ferguson et al., "Expert Declaration of Dr. Stephen B. Levine in Support of Plaintiff's Motion for Preliminary Injunction," United States District Court, Western District of Washington at Tacoma, Civil No. 3:21- cv-5359. *See also:* "The Effect of Puberty Blockers on the Accrual of Bone Mass," *Society for Evidence-Based Gender Medicine*, May 1, 2021, segm.org/the_effect_of_puberty_blockers_on_the_accrual_of_bone_mass; Sanchez Manning, "Puberty Blockers Given to Children Who Say They Were Born in the Wrong Body and Want to 'Change Gender' May Lower Their' IQs," *Daily Mail*, January 13, 2024, www.dailymail.co.uk/news/article-12960869/Puberty-blockers-given-children-say-born-wrong-body-want-change-gender-lower-IQs.html.

Black box puberty blocker FDA warning due to brain swelling and vision loss: "Risk of Pseudotumor Cerebri Added to Labeling for Gonadotropin-Releasing Hormone Agonists," press release, American Academy of Pediatrics, July 1, 2022, www.fda.gov/media/159663/download.

30   *The Dutch protocol:* Maria A. T. C. van der Loos, MD, et al., "Children and Adolescents in the Amsterdam Cohort of Gender Dysphoria: Trends in Diagnostic and Treatment Trajectories During the First 20 years of the Dutch Protocol," *Journal of Sexual Medicine*, January 26, 2023, doi.org/10.1093/jsxmed/qdac029.

Michael Biggs analysis of flaws in the Dutch protocol: M. Biggs, "The Dutch Protocol for Juvenile Transsexuals: Origins and Evidence," *Journal of Sex & Marital Therapy*, September 19, 2022, doi.org/10.1080/0092623X.2022.2121238.

32   *Little evidence that childhood-onset is persistent:* Alex Byrne, "Another Myth of Persistence?" *Archives of Sexual Behavior*, June 17, 2024, doi.org/10.1007/s10508-024-03005-1.

33   *Gender identity orders were rare until recently:* "Prevalence," *The Diagnostic and Statistical Manual of Mental Disorders*, 5th ed. (DSM–5), "Gender Dysphoria" chapter, 454.

Almost all kids on puberty blockers go on to cross-sex hormones: Maria A. T. C. van der Loos, MD, et al., "Continuation of Gender-Affirming Hormones in Transgender People Starting Puberty Suppression in Adolescence: A Cohort Study in the Netherlands," *Lancet*, December

2022, doi.org/10.1016/S2352-4642(22)00254-1.

Analysis of children seeking treatment for gender confusion: Robin Respaut and Chad Terhune, "Number of Transgender Children Seeking Treatment Surges in U.S.," *Reuters* October 6, 2022, www.reuters.com/article/usa-transyouth-data/number-of-transgender-children-seeking-treatment-surges-in-u-s-idINL1N3142UU/.

Wright MD et al., "National Estimates of Gender-Affirming Surgery."

Kaiser's share of health care in states: "Market Share and Enrollment of Largest Three Insurers—Large Group Market," Kaiser Family Foundation, www.kff.org/other/state-indicator/market-share-and-enrollment-of-largest-three-insurers-large-group-market/?currentTimeframe=0&sortModel=%7B%22colId%22:%22Location%22,%22sort%22:%22asc%22%7D.

*Indicates pseudonym.

34   *Effects of supplemental estrogen on males:* Lauren Schwartz et al., "Emerging and Accumulating Safety Signals for the Use of Estrogen among Transgender Women," *Discover Mental Health*, June 12, 2025. *See also*: Jason van Heesewijk et al., "Cognitive Functioning after Long-Term Gender-Affirming Hormone Therapy—a study in Older Transgender Individuals," 5th EPath Conference, Endocrinology, Transgender Health, April 27, 2023, epath2023.exordo.com/programme/presentation/98.

34–35 *Supplemental testosterone's effects females, extreme vaginal atrophy and dryness:* M Baldasarre et al., "Effects of Long-Term High Dose Testosterone Administration on Vaginal Epithelium Structure and Estrogen Receptor-α and -β Expression of Young Women," *Nature Portfolio*, September 2013, doi:10.1038/ijir.2013.9.

Increased risk of cardiovascular disease: Talal Alzahrani, MD, et al., "Cardiovascular Disease Risk Factors and Myocardial Infarction in the Transgender Population," *Circulation: Cardiovascular Quality and Outcomes*, April 5, 2019, doi:10.1161/CIRCOUTCOMES.119.005597.

Increased liver cancer risk: Daniel Martin, "Doctors Admit Link between Transgender Hormone Therapy and Cancer in Leaked Emails," *Telegraph*, March 5, 2024, www.telegraph.co.uk/news/2024/03/05/wpath-tansgender-hormone-therapy-cancer-links-leaked-emails/.

Lyvia Maria Bezerra da Silva et al., "Pelvic Floor Dysfunction in Transgender Men on Gender-Affirming Hormone Therapy: A Descriptive Cross-Sectional Study," *Int Urogynecology*, May 2024, doi:10.1007/s00192-024-05779-3. *See also*: "Information on Testosterone Hormone Therapy," *USCF Transgender Care*, March 2025, transcare.ucsf. edu/article/information-testosterone-hormone-therapy.

35   Helena Kerschner testimony to the Florida Board of Medicine and Florida Board of Osteopathic Medicine, video uploaded by Thoughts on Things and Stuff, October 28, 2022, www.youtube.com/ watch?v=ZfbiS_vdXco.
        *Indicates pseudonym

36   Leslie McClurg, "Transgender and Non-Binary People Are Up to Six Times More Likely to Have Autism," *NPR*, January 15, 2023, https:// www.npr.org/2023/01/15/1149318664/transgender-and-non-binary-people-are-up-to-six-times-more-likely-to-have-autism.
        Jonathon W. Wonta et al., "Mental Health Diagnoses Among Transgender Patients in the Clinical Setting: An All-Payer Electronic Health Record Study," *Transgender Health*, November 2019, doi:10.1089/ trgh.2019.0029.

37–39   Author interview with Stephanie Winn.
        Bret Weinstein and Heather Heying, *Dark Horse* podcast, March 27, 2021, www.youtube.com/watch?v=TfV-Hg26Q-U.

39–42   Author interview with "Carol."

42   Detrans Reddit: https://www.reddit.com/r/detrans/.

43   *Experts: "gender affirmation" can act as conversion therapy:* K. Zucker, "Debate: Different Strokes for Different Folks," *Child and Adolescent Mental Health*, May 31, 2019, doi:10.1111/camh.12330, and *Tingley vs. Ferguson* et al., "Expert Declaration of Dr. Stephen B. Levine." *Kristina Olson's statistical analysis reevaluated and found flawed:* Walter R. Schumm, PhD, and Duane W. Crawford, PhD, "Is Research on Transgender Children What It Seems? Comments on Recent Research on Transgender Children with High Levels of Parental Support," *Linacre Quarterly*, November 2019, doi:10.1177/002436391988479.

Chapter Two: Consent to This "Care" . . . or Else

44   Author interview with Jamie Reed.

45   Anne P. Haas, PhD, Philip L. Rogers, PhD, and Jody L. Herman, "Suicide Attempts among Transgender and Gender Non-Conforming Adults," American Foundation for Suicide Prevention and the Williams Institute UCLA School of Law, January 2014, williamsinstitute. law.ucla.edu/wp-content/uploads/Trans-GNC-Suicide-Attempts-Jan-2014.pdf.

46   Jody L. Herman, et al, "Suicide Thoughts and Attempts among Trans-
         gender Adults: Findings from the 2015 U.S. Transgender Survey,"
         Williams Institute UCLA School of Law, 2019, williamsinstitute.law.
         ucla.edu/wp-content/uploads/Suicidality-Transgender-Sep-2019.
         pdf.

46–47   *Finland study:* Sami Matti Ruuska et al., "All-Cause and Suicide Mor-
         talities among Adolescents and Young Adults Who Contacted Special-
         ised Gender Identity Services in Finland in 1996–2019" *BMJ Mental
         Health*, February 16, 2024, doi.org/10.1136/bmjment-2023-300940.

47   *19x suicide rate after genital surgery:* Cecelia Dhejne et al., "Long-Term
         Follow-Up of Transsexual Persons Undergoing Sex Reassignment
         Surgery: Cohort Study in Sweden," *PLOS One*, February 22, 2011, doi.
         org/10.1371/journal.pone.0016885.

47–48   Michael Biggs, "Suicide by Clinic-Referred Transgender Adolescents
         in the United Kingdom," *Archives of Sexual Behavior,* January 18, 2022,
         doi.org/10.1007/s10508-022-02287-7.

48–49   E. Colemen et al., "Standards of Care for the Health of Transgender
         and Gender Diverse People, Version 8," World Professional Associa-
         tion for Transgender Health (WPATH), September 15, 2022, doi.org/
         10.1080/26895269.2022.2100644; "Mission," WPATH, www.wpath.
         org/media/cms/Documents/SOC%20v7/SOC%20V7_English.pdf;
         "FAQs," WPATH, www.wpath.org/media/cms/Documents/SOC%20
         v8/SOC-8%20FAQs%20-%20WEBSITE2.pdf (last accessed 2024).

49   *Claims that gender procedures are life-saving/ medically necessary:*
         American Psychological Association, www.apa.org/topics/lgbtq/gen-
         der-affirmative-care (last accessed 2024).
         Endocrine Society: www.endocrine.org/news-and-advocacy/news-
         room/2023/ama-gender-affirming-care (last accessed 2024).
         American Medical Association: www.ama-assn.org/press-center/
         press-releases/ama-reinforces-opposition-restrictions-transgen-
         der-medical-care (last accessed 2024).
         "Rachel" Levine, post by @HHS_ASH, February 24, 2022, x.com/
         HHS_ASH/status/1496862186664341505.
         Seattle Children's Hospital: publications.aap.org/pediatrics/article-ab-
         stract/153/1/e2023064292/196236/Prohibition-of-Gender-Affirm-
         ing-Care-as-a-Form-of? (last accessed 2024).
         *Medical associations that have made statements in support of medical and
         surgical interventions on minors:* glaad.org/medical-association-state-
         ments-supporting-trans-youth-healthcare-and-against-discriminato-
         ry/ (last accessed 2024).

50   *Tavistock GIDS:* Hannah Barnes, *Time to Think: The Inside Story of the Collapse of the Tavistock's Gender Service for Children* (Swift Press 2023).

51   "Keira Bell: My Story," *Persuasion*, April 7, 2021, www.persuasion. community/p/keira-bell-my-story.

52   *The Cass Review:* cass.independent-review.uk/home/publications/final-report/.

53   Hilary Cass, BBC interview, April 20, 2024, www.bbc.com/news/health-68863594.

Dr. Ben Hoffman, "Statement From the American Academy of Pediatrics," May 8, 2024, threadreaderapp.com/thread/1788200424236843097.html.

Endocrine Society, "Statement in Support of Gender-Affirming Care," May 8, 2024, www.endocrine.org/news-and-advocacy/newsroom/2024/statement-in-support-of-gender-affirming-care.

WPATH response to Cass Review: www.wpath.org/media/cms/Documents/Public%20Policies/2024/17.05.24%20Response%20Cass%20Review%20FINAL%20with%20ed%20note.pdf.

54   *Finland pulls back on youth gender procedures:* segm.org/sites/default/files/Finnish_Guidelines_2020_Minors_Unofficial%20Translation.pdf.

55   *Sweden response, teen trans procedures:* Richard Orange, "Teenage Transgender Row Splits Sweden as Dysphoria Diagnoses Soar by 1,500%," *Guardian*, February 22, 2020, www.theguardian.com/society/2020/feb/22/ssweden-teenage-transgender-row-dysphoria-diagnoses-soar. *See also:* SEGM, "Summary of Key Recommendations from the Swedish National Board of Health and Welfare," Febrauary 22, 2022, segm.org/segm-summary-sweden-prioritizes-therapy-curbs-hormones-for-gender-dysphoric-youth.

Sweden, France, and Norway raise alarms on "transitioning" minors: "Expert Report of James Cantor, PhD, " *Boe v. Marshall*, Case 2:22-cv-00184-LCB-CWB, Document 557–2.

WPATH Standards of Care: E. Colemen et al., "Standards of Care for the Health of Transgender and Gender Diverse People, Version 8," World Professional Association for Transgender Health (WPATH), September 15, 2022, doi.org/10.1080/26895269.2022.2100644.

Emails, Johns Hopkins: WPATH is suppressing their systematic review research done on WPATH's behalf: "Exhibit 167," *Boe v. Marshall*, Case 2:22-cv-00184-LCB-CWB, Document 560, May 27, 2024.

WPATH denied Johns Hopkins the ability to publish: ibid.

American Academy of Pediatrics' ultimatum to WPATH: "Expert Report of James Cantor, PhD, " *Boe v. Marshall*, Case 2:22-cv-00184-LCB-CWB, Document 557–2.

56–57   *Draft minimum ages in WPATH SOC 8:* Jennifer Block, "US Transgender Health Guidelines Leave Age of Treatment Initiation Open to Clinical Judgment," *BMJ*, September 27, 2022, dx.doi.org/10.1136/bmj.o2303.

Double mastectomy at 13: Peter Suratos, "Kaiser Permanente sued over hormone therapy," *NBC Bay Area*, February 24, 2023, www.nbcbayarea.com/news/local/kaiser-permanente-sued-over-hormone-therapy/3164935/. *See also*: Christina Buttons, "BREAKING: Second Lawsuit Filed in US Against Medical Transition of Minors," *Reality's Last Stand*, June 14, 2023, www.realityslaststand.com/p/breaking-second-lawsuit-filed-in.

57   Top surgery risks, complications, and side-effects: Fan Liang, MD, "Top Surgery (Chest Feminization or Chest Masculinization)," *Johns Hopkins Medicine*, www.hopkinsmedicine.org/health/treatment-tests-and-therapies/top-surgery (last accessed July 2025).

57–58   "Phalloplasty Risks and Complications," *Phallo.net*, www.phallo.net/risks-complications/ (last accessed July 2025).

Dr. Gabriel Del Corral, "I tell all my patients that the complication rate for Phalloplasty can be 100%." Ibid.

Description and images of procedure: Mamoon Rashid and Muhammad Sarmad Tamimy, "Phalloplasty: The Dream and the Reality," *Indian Plastic Surgery*, 2013, doi:10.4103/0970-0358.118606.

58–59   "Vaginoplasty," Cleveland Clinic, 2024, my.clevelandclinic.org/health/procedures/21572-vaginoplasty.

Vaginoplasty using colon causes fistulas, other complications: Wouter B van der Sluis et al., "Neovaginal Discharge in Transgender Women after Vaginoplasty: A Diagnostic and Treatment Algorithm," *International Journal Transgender Health*, February 13, 2020 doi:10.1080/26895269.2020.1725710.

More than half WPATH physicians performed vaginoplasty on minors: Christine Milrod, PhD, and Dan H. Karasic, MD, "Age Is Just a Number: WPATH-Affiliated Surgeons' Experiences and Attitudes Toward Vaginoplasty in Transgender Females Under 18 Years of Age in the United States," *Journal of Sexual Medicine*, March 19, 2017, doi.org/10.1016/j.jsxm.2017.02.007.

Chapter Three: The Media and the Message

60   Azeen Ghorayshi, "Biden Officials Pushed to Remove Age Limits for Trans Surgery, Documents Show," *New York Times,* June 25, 2024, www.nytimes.com/2024/06/25/health/transgender-minors-surgeries.html.

New York Times op-ed mentioning Rachel Levine's pressure to remove age minimums: Pamela Paul, "Why Is the U.S. Still Pretending We Know Gender-Affirming Care Works?" *New York Times,* July 12, 2024, www.nytimes.com/2024/07/12/opinion/gender-affirming-care-cass-review.html.

Washington Post article on Rachel Levine's pressure to remove WPATH age minimums: Megan McArdle, "The Crucial Questions about Gender Care Are Not Political or Legal," *Washington Post,* July 2, 2024, www.washingtonpost.com/opinions/2024/07/02/transgender-medicine-scientific-legal-political-children/.

61   *GLAAD press release on anti-LGBTQ laws:* "States Legislators Propose 300 Anti-LGBTQ Bills as GLAAD Releases Updated Reporter Guide, Resources," February 9, 2023, glaad.org/releases/state-legislators-propose-300-anti-lgbtq-bills-glaad-releases-updated-reporter-guide/.

MAP press release: "Under Fire Series: The War on LGBTQ People in America," www.mapresearch.org/under-fire-report (last accessed July 2025).

Human Rights Campaign press release: Brandon Wolf, "HRC's Weekly State Fights Report: Slew of Anti-LGBTQ+ Bills Become Law," March 26, 2024, www.hrc.org/press-releases/hrcs-weekly-state-fights-report-slew-of-anti-lgbtq-bills-become-law.

Annette Choi, "Record Number of Anti-LGBTQ Bills Were Introduced in 2023," *CNN,* January 22, 2024, CNN: www.cnn.com/politics/anti-lgbtq-plus-state-bill-rights-dg/index.html.

Jo Yurcaba, "From Drag Bans to Sports Restrictions, 75 Anti-LGBTQ Bills Have Become Law in 2023," *NBC,* December 17, 2023, www.nbcnews.com/nbc-out/out-politics-and-policy/75-anti-lgbtq-bills-become-law-2023-rcna124250.

Kaleigh Rogers and Mary Radcliffe, "Over 100 Anti-LGBTQ+ Laws Passed in the Last Five Years," *FiveThirtyEight,* May 25, 2023, fivethirtyeight.com/features/anti-lgbtq-laws-red-states/.

"More Than 275 Bills Targeting LGBTQ Rights Flood State Legislatures": Nick Robertson, *Hill,* January 16, 2024, thehill.com/homenews/lgbtq/4412024-state-legislatures-bills-targeting-lgbtq-rights/.

"These 5 States Are Doing the Most to Target LGBTQ People": *Rolling Stone*, July 15, 2023, www.rollingstone.com/culture/culture-features/worst-anti-lgbtq-states-america-trans-legislation-1234788961/.

"Wave of Anti-LGBTQ Laws Passed Across Country," *CBS News*, June 28, 2023, www.cbsnews.com/video/wave-of-anti-lgbtq-laws-passed-across-country/.

Kacen Bayless and Jonathan Shorman, "'I'm Terrified.' Missouri Lawmakers File Onslaught of Anti-LGBTQ Bills for 2024 Session," *Kansas City Star*, March 22, 2024, www.kansascity.com/news/politics-government/article282969448.html.

Orion Rummler, "House Republicans Are Adding Dozens of Anti-LGBTQ+ Measures to Must-Pass Bills," *19th News*, August 8, 2023, 19thnews.org/2023/08/house-republicans-anti-lgbtq-measures-federal-spending-bills/.

Susan Miller, "'War' on LGBTQ Existence: 8 Ways the Record Onslaught of 650 Bills Targets the Community," *USA Today*, March 31, 2023, www.usatoday.com/story/news/nation/2023/03/31/650-anti-lgbtq-bills-introduced-us/11552357002/.

63   Stephen W. Thrasher, "The Vital Need for Queer Studies," *Inside Higher Education*, September 6, 2018, www.insidehighered.com/advice/2018/09/07/queer-studies-benefit-journalism-education-and-education-general-opinion.

Anna Marks, "Ohio Is about to Make Queer Kids Miserable," *New York Times*, December 31, 2024, www.nytimes.com/live/2025/01/02/opinion/thepoint#ohio-queer-kids-legislation.

65   *PRRI poll 2022:* "Americans' Support for Key LGBTQ Rights Continues to Tick Upward," *PRRI*, March 17, 2022, www.prri.org/research/americans-support-for-key-lgbtq-rights-continues-to-tick-upward/.

PRRI poll 2023: "Views on LGBTQ Rights in All 50 States: Findings from PRRI's 2023 American Values Atlas," March 12, 2024, www.prri.org/research/views-on-lgbtq-rights-in-all-50-states/.

66   Jesse Singal, "Why Is the Same Misleading Language about Youth Gender Medicine Copied and Pasted into Dozens of CNN.com Articles?" *Singal-Minded*, March 22, 2024, jessesingal.substack.com/p/why-is-the-same-misleading-language.

Tara John, "England's Health Service to Stop Prescribing Puberty Blockers to Transgender Kids," *CNN*, March 13, 2024, www.cnn.com/2024/03/13/uk/england-nhs-puberty-blockers-trans-children-intl-gbr/index.html.

67　　　Jenavieve Hatch, "A Mom of a Nonbinary Teen Became an Anti-Trans Activist, Fracturing a California Family," *Sacramento Bee*, April 10, 2024, www.sacbee.com/news/local/article285961211.html#storylink =cpy.

68–75　Author interview with Beth Bourne (chapter segment adapted from Anita Bartholomew, "When Media Promote the Cult's Narrative," *Good Question*, April 17, 2024, anitabartholomew.substack.com/p/ when-media-promote-the-cults-narrative.

72　　　Jesse Singal, "When Children Say They're Trans," *Atlantic*, July–August 2018, www.theatlantic.com/magazine/archive/2018/07/when-a-child-says-shes-trans/561749/.

74　　　Parents With Inconvenient Truths About Trans (PITT), www.pittparents.com/.

　　　　Newsweek article about Beth Bourne: Robert C. Bulman, "Because 'Moms for Hate' Just Doesn't Have the Same Ring," *Newsweek*, July 11, 2024, www.newsweek.com/because-moms-hate-just-doesnt-have-same-ring-opinion-1923855.

　　　　Hannah Holzer, "Why Is UC Davis Letting a Raging Transphobe Continue to Work around Students?" *Sacramento Bee*, June 30, 2024, www.sacbee.com/opinion/article289560160.html#storylink=cpy.

　　　　Elisa Bourne, Davis School Board meeting, January 19, 2023, davis. granicus.com/player/clip/1517?view_id=4.

Chapter Four: Today's Lesson: Reject Your Sex

77　　　*Williams Institute 2017 estimates, 13- to 17-year-olds who believed themselves to be transgender:* Herman et al., "Age of Individuals Who identify as Transgender in the United States," 2.

　　　　Williams Institute 2022 estimates, 13 to 17-year-olds who believed themselves to be transgender: Herman et al., "How Many Adults and Youth Identify as Transgender in the United States?," 1.

　　　　Teens in New York vs Wyoming who identify as the opposite sex: ibid., 9.

　　　　CDC survey finds 5.5% of high schoolers say they're trans or think they might be: Nicolas A. Suarez, MPH, et al., "Disparities in School Connectedness, Unstable Housing, Experiences of Violence, Mental Health, and Suicidal Thoughts and Behaviors Among Transgender and Cisgender High School Students—Youth Risk Behavior Survey," US Department of Health and Human Services, Centers for Disease Control and Prevention, MMWR Supplement, October 10, 2024.

8% of Oregon students gender-confused: Colt Gill, Director of Oregon Department of Education, in an interview with Dave Miller, "Think Out Loud," *Oregon Public Broadcasting,* April 21, 2022, www.opb.org/article/2022/04/21/support-for-transgender-students-in-oregon-schools-goes-beyond-salem-keizer/.

9.2% of students in one Pittsburgh school district gender-confused: Kacie M. Kidd, MD, "Prevalence of Gender-Diverse Youth in an Urban School District," *Pediatrics,* June 2021, doi.org/10.1542/peds.2020-049823.

Rapid onset gender dysphoria: Littman, "Parent Reports of Adolescents and Young Adults."

Other social contagions: Stephen Allison et al., "Anorexia Nervosa and Social Contagion: Clinical Implications," *Australian & New Zealand Journal of Psychiatry,* August 22, 2013, doi.org/10.1177/0004867413502.

Dorothy E Grice and Cathy L Budman, "Tics and Tic-Like Behaviors: Social Contagion in Pandemic Times," *Journal of the American Academy of Child & Adolescent Psychiatry,* October 12, 2022, doi: 10.1016/j.jaac.2022.07.332.

John D. Haltigan et al., "Social Media as an Incubator of Personality and Behavioral Psychopathology: Symptom and Disorder Authenticity or Psychosomatic Social Contagion?" *Comprehensive Psychiatry,* February 2023, doi.org/10.1016/j.comppsych.2022.152362.

Lawrence Patihis, PhD, "Social Contagions and Iatrogenic Harms in Psychology," *Lawrence Patihis' Substack,* April 8, 2024, lawrencepatihis.substack.com/p/social-contagions-and-iatrogenic.

Recovered false memories: Ethan Watters, "The Forgotten Lessons of the Recovered Memory Movement," *New York Times,* September 27, 2022, www.nytimes.com/2022/09/27/opinion/recovered-memory-therapy-mental-health.html.

79   *Queer theory comprehensive sex ed rejects "cis-heteronormative framework":* Hannah Dyer et al., "Queer Futurity and Childhood Innocence: Beyond the Injury of Development," *Global Studies of Childhood,* October 9, 2016, doi.org/10.1177/2043610616671056.

80–81   "The Future of Sex Education," www.futureofsexed.org (last accessed July 2025).

State sex-ed requirements: "State Profiles, *SIECUS,* 2025, siecus.org/siecus-state-profiles/.

Advocates for Youth, Answer Sex Ed Honestly, SIECUS, "National Sex Education Standards," Future of Sex Education Initiative, www.advocatesforyouth.org/wp-content/uploads/2021/11/NSES-2020-web-updated2.pdf (last updated 2020).

81   *Foucault:* Nicholas L. Syrett, "Introduction to 'Sex across the Ages': Restoring Intergenerational Dynamics to Queer History,'" *Berghahn Journals*, March 1, 2020, doi.org/10.3167/hrrh.2020.460101.

82   Pat Califia, "The Age of Consent: The Great Kiddie Porn Panic of '77,'" www.ipce.info/ipceweb/Library/califa_aoc_frame.htm.
        Rubin calls for liberating deviants as "sexual minorities": Gayle S. Rubin, "Thinking Sex: Notes for a Radical Theory of the Politics of Sexuality," in *Pleasure and Danger: Exploring Female Sexuality*, ed. Carol S. Vance (Routledge & Kegan Paul 1984), 143–179.

83   Kathy Rudy, "LGBTQ . . . Z?" *Hypatia*, Summer 2012, www.jstor.org/stable/23254843.

84   Brooke Migdon, "Earmark for Philly LGBTQ Center Pulled over 'Kink' Parties," *Hill*, March 6, 2024, thehill.com/homenews/lgbtq/4513710-earmark-pulled-philly-lgbtq-center-kink-parties/.
        Rochelle Olson, "Legal Experts Say Change to Minnesota Human Rights Act Won't Protect Pedophiles," *Minnesota Star Tribune*, May 18, 2023, www.startribune.com/legal-experts-say-change-to-minnesota-human-rights-act-wont-protect-pedophiles/600275868.

85   *LGBTQ holidays:* "LGBTQ Community Calendar," *GLAAD*, www.startribune.com/legal-experts-say-change-to-minnesota-human-rights-act-wont-protect-pedophiles/600275868.
        Teny Sahakian, "LA Elementary Schools to Celebrate National Coming Out Day with a Week of LGBTQ+ Lessons," *Fox 11 Los Angeles*, October 9, 2023, www.foxla.com/news/los-angeles-elementary-schools-celebrate-national-coming-out-day-lgbtq-lessons.
        "Happy Pride Month from Chicago Public Schools," video uploaded by Chicago Public Schools, June 11, 2021, www.youtube.com/watch?v=Ws7iV6ewhLg.
        Portland Elementary School Pride event: @LarsLarsonShow, post on X.com, May 1, 2023, twitter.com/LarsLarsonShow/status/1653097970395652097.

86   Author interview with Grace Ellison, pseudonym.
        Author interview with Raef Haggag.
        Robin Stevenson, *Pride Puppy!* (Orca Book Publishers 2024).
        DeShanna Neal and Trinity Neal, *My Rainbow* (Kokila 2020).
        Charlotte Sullivan Wild, *Love, Violet* (Farrar, Straus and Giroux 2022).

87   Author interview with Erica Anderson, PhD.
        Author interview with David Habib Martin, LPD.
        Katherine Locke, *What Are Your Words? A Book about Pronouns* (Little, Brown Books for Young Readers 2021).

88   Author interview with Stephanie Winn, LMFT.
      Sarah Hoffman and Ian Hoffman, *Jacob's Room to Choose* (Magination Press 2019).
      DeShanna Neal and Trinity Neal, *My Rainbow* (Kokila 2020).

90   *Montgomery schools teachers and principals object to "Pride" curriculum:* Declaration of Robert McCaw, *Mahmoud v. McKnight*, Case 8:23-cv-01380-DLB Document 47-1.

91   Theresa Thorn, *It Feels Good to Be Yourself: A Book about Gender Identity* (Henry Holt and Co. 2019).

92   "HiTOPS' Org Sneaks Sexual & LGBTQ+ Curriculum into Schools, Goal to Strip Parental Opt-Out Rights," video uploaded by Project Veritas, September 13, 2023, www.youtube.com/watch?v=t1tTtc4Q-24.
      "Part 2: HiTOPS Designs Sexual Identity Training for Kindergartners," video uploaded by Project Veritas, September 20, 2023, www.youtube.com/watch?v=Ds8VAtOXRbU.
      Erin Lee's daughter and the secret GSA "art" club: Gender & Sexuality Art Club, video uploaded by Independence Institute TV, May 8, 2022, www.youtube.com/watch?v=CLjmE7GhsHI.

93   Abigail Shrier, "How Activist Teachers Recruit Kids," *Truth Fairy*, November 18, 2021, www.thetruthfairy.info/p/how-activist-teachers-recruit-kids.

94   *Jessica Konen sues school:* Josh Kopitch, "Spreckels Union School District Settles with Parent over Indoctrination Allegations," *KSBW Action News*, August 29, 2023, www.ksbw.com/article/spreckels-union-school-district-settles-with-parent-over-indoctrination-allegations/44942724.
      Author interview with Dr. Erica Anderson.
      "Expert Affidavit of Dr. Stephen B. Levine," *P.F., B.F., P.W., and S.W. v. Kettle Moraine School District*, Case 2021CV001650 Document 78, Filed 02-03-2023.

Chapter Five: Watch Out Kids, Your Parents Aren't "Safe"

96   Author interview with Kim Zucker
      *Indicates pseudonym.

98   *Trans influencers persuades kids to run away:* "The Runaway," *Parents With Inconvenient Truths About Trans*, January 27, 2023, www.pittparents.com/p/the-runaway?utm_source=publication-search; see *also:* "This Is How They Are Stealing Our Children," *Parents With Inconvenient*

Truths About Trans, July 15, 2024, www.pittparents.com/p/this-is-how-they-are-stealing-our; and "Estrangement Survey: Managing Your Response to a No-Contact Minor Or Adult Child," *Parents With Inconvenient Truths About Trans*, December 21, 2022, www.pittparents.com/p/estrangement-survey-managing-your?utm_source=publication-search. Author interview with Erin Friday.
*Names and identifying details changed.

106   *Sage Blair:* "Complaint," *Blair v. Appomattox*, Case 6:23-cv-00047-NKM Document 1, August 22, 2023.

107   "Plaintiff's Brief in Opposition to Defendant Appomattox County School Board's Motion To Dismiss," *Blair v. Appomattox*, Case 6:23-cv-00047-NKM Document 50, October 16, 2023; *see also:* "The Saga of Sage," *Parents With Inconvenient Truths About Trans*, May 5, 2022, pitt.substack.com/p/saga-of-sage.
        Olympia schools: Author interview with Alesha Perkins.

108–116 Author interviews with anonymous parents and teachers; emails and other records obtained via public records requests by anonymous sources.
        *Names and identifying details changed

116   "Trans Minors Protected from Parents under Washington Law," *KNKX Public Radio*, May 9, 2023, www.knkx.org/law/2023-05-09/trans-minors-protected-from-parents-under-washington-law.

Chapter Six: Watch Out Parents: No One, Nowhere, and Nothing Is Safe

117–120 Author interview with Jamie Reed.

120   *Losing custody for not transing kids:* Madalaine Elhabbal,"Fathers Who Lost Their Children to Gender Ideology: 'I Feel So Betrayed,'" *Catholic News Agency*, December 7, 2024, www.catholicnewsagency.com/news/260903/fathers-who-lost-their-children-to-gender-ideology-i-feel-so-betrayed.
        "CA Father Fights for 3-Year-Old Son Forced to Live 'Non-Binary' Life By Mother," *California Family Council*, August 11,2023, www.californiafamily.org/2023/08/ca-father-fights-for-3-year-old-son-forced-to-live-non-binary-life-by-mother/https://www.becketlaw.org/case/m-c-and-j-c-v-indiana-department-of-child-services/.
        Caitlin Tilley, "New York Father Loses Legal Battle to Stop His Son, 8, from Taking Puberty Blockers to Change Gender," *Daily Mail*, February 2, 2024, www.dailymail.co.uk/health/article-13030699/gen-

der-transition-custody-battle.html.

121   Tierin-Rose Mandelburg, "Father Details Losing Custody Battle over 2-Year-Old's Gender Transition," *mrcTV*, December 18, 2023, www.mrctv.org/blog/tierin-rose-mandelburg/father-details-losing-custody-battle-over-2-year-olds-gender-transition.
       Google search on "gender-affirming" and "life-saving": tiny.cc/qfe6zz.
       Heather Boerner, "What the Science on Gender-Affirming Care for Transgender Kids Really Shows," *Scientific American*, May 12, 2022, www.scientificamerican.com/article/what-the-science-on-gender-affirming-care-for-transgender-kids-really-shows/.

122   Steve Mirsky, "175 Years of *Scientific American*: The Good, the Bad, and the Debunking," *Scientific American*, August 29, 2020, www.scientificamerican.com/podcast/episode/175-years-of-scientific-american-the-good-the-bad-and-the-debunking/.
       Elizabeth Mondegreen, "Detransitioner Files Lawsuit Against 'Gender-Affirming' Clinicians," *Unherd*, October 23, 2023, unherd.com/newsroom/detransitioner-files-lawsuit-against-gender-affirming-clinicians/.

123   Robbie Feinberg, "Maine Expands Ability of Older Teens to Receive Gender-Affirming Care Without Parents' Consent," *Maine Public*, July 12, 2023, www.mainepublic.org/politics/2023-07-12/maine-expands-ability-of-older-teens-to-receive-gender-affirming-care-without-parents-consent.
       Minnesota: "Minor's Consent for Healthcare," *MN House Research*, August 2023, https://www.house.mn.gov/hrd/pubs/ss/ssminorhc.pdf.
       Author interview with Erin Friday.
       "Trans Minors Protected from Parents under Washington Law," *KNKX Public Radio*, May 9, 2023, www.knkx.org/law/2023-05-09/trans-minors-protected-from-parents-under-washington-law.
       Amanda Hernández, "More Blue States Declare Themselves Sanctuaries for Transgender Health Care," *Stateline*, June 22, 2023, stateline.org/2023/06/22/more-blue-states-declare-themselves-sanctuaries-for-transgender-health-care/.
       Author interview with Jamie Reed.

124   "The Numbers," *ROGD Boys*, www.rogdboys.org/the-numbers.
       Parents With Inconvenient Truths About Trans teleconference on ROGD boy, unrecorded, September 2023.

125–131 Author interview with Ellie.
       *Names and certain other identifying information changed.

132–136 Author interview with Jeannette Cooper.

Chapter Seven: Is Transgender Actually a Thing (and Is It Just One Thing)?

137   "Information on Testosterone Hormone Therapy," *USCF Transgender Care*, March 2025, transcare.ucsf.edu/article/information-testosterone-hormone-therapy.

138–145 Author interview with Claire.
        *Names and certain other identifying information changed.

143   "Accurate Transition Regret and Detransition Rates Are Unknown," *Society for Evidence-Based Gender Medicine*, September 11, 2023, segm.org/regret-detransition-rate-unknown.

144   Aida Cerundolo and Carrie Mendoza, "How US Billing Rules Make Detransitioning a Hotel California Nightmare," *New York Post*, June 14, 2023, nypost.com/2023/06/14/how-us-billing-rules-make-detransitioning-a-hotel-california-nightmare/.

145   Genny Beemyn, "Colleges and Universities That Cover Transition-Related Medical Expenses under Student Health Insurance," *Campus Pride*, July 27, 2024, www.campuspride.org/tpc/student-health-insurance/.

146   *Only about 25% of men claiming to be women are same-sex attracted:* Bailey and Blanchard, "Gender Dysphoria Is Not One Thing."
        Blanchard on AGPs denial that they are AGP: Louise Perry, "What Is Autogynephilia?" an interview with Dr. Ray Blanchard, November 6, 2019, quillette.com/2019/11/06/what-is-autogynephilia-an-interview-with-dr-ray-blanchard/.

147   Author interview with Ray Blanchard.
        AGP's post about what it feels like to be attracted to oneself: @RayAlexWilliams, post on X, March 6, 2024, x.com/RayAlexWilliams/status/1765376122701611049.

148   *Transvestic fetishism:* See the discussion on "transvestic disorder in the "Paraphilic Disorders" chapter of the *The Diagnostic and Statistical Manual of Mental Disorders* (5th ed.; DSM–5) (American Psychiatric Association, 2013). Also see the "Gender Dysphoria" chapter.

149   *Swedish paper on transvestic fetishists:* Niklas Långström and Kenneth J. Zucker, "Transvestic Fetishism in the General Population," *Journal of Sex & Marital Therapy*, March–April 2005, doi.org/10.1080/00926230590477934.
        Deceptive behavior in cross-dressing straight males: Kenneth J. Zucker et al., "Demographics, Behavior Problems, and Psychosexual Characteristics of Adolescents with Gender Identity Disorder or Transvestic Fetishism," *Journal of Sex & Marital Therapy*, March 5, 2012, doi.org/1

0.1080/0092623X.2011.611219.

Reduxx reports, sex crimes, cross-dressing men: Genevieve Gluck, "Exclusive Details: Norwegian Trans-Identified Men Charged with Gang Rape of Young Girl," *Reduxx*, January 13, 2025, reduxx.info/exclusive-details-norwegian-trans-identified-men-charged-with-gang-rape-of-young-girl/. *See also:* Anna Slatz, "Exclusive: Transgender Pedophile Given Lenient Sentence for Sexually Abusing His 5-Year-Old Daughter After Court Considers 'Transphobia' in Sentence," *Reduxx*, January 16, 2025, reduxx.info/exclusive-transgender-pedophile-given-lenient-sentence-for-sexually-abusing-his-5-year-old-daughter-after-court-considers-transphobia-in-sentence/; and "Brazil: Trans Activist Day Care Worker Arrested for Sexual Abuse of Six Young Children," *Reduxx*, July 3, 2025, reduxx.info/brazil-trans-activist-day-care-worker-arrested-for-sexual-abuse-of-six-young-children/.

Ramon Antonio Vargas, "Dylan Mulvaney Says Woman-of-the-Year Award 'Means So Much More' after Bud Light Backlash, *Guardian*, October 14, 2023, www.theguardian.com/world/2023/oct/13/us-tiktok-trans-activist-woman-of-the-year-award-bud-light-boycott.

See also, more male women of the year: Alec Schemmel, "Transgender Lawmaker Honored on *USA Today* 'Women of the Year' Llist," *ABC News 4*, March 20, 2023, abcnews4.com/news/nation-world/transgender-lawmaker-honored-on-usa-today-women-of-the-year-list-leigh-finke-minneasota-rachel-levine-lgbtq.

See also, more male women of the year: Allison Bloom, "Geena Rocero Honored as One of Glamour's 2023 Women of the Year!" *GLAAD*, November 1, 2023, glaad.org/geena-rocero-honored-as-one-of-glamours-2023-women-of-the-year/.

Abby Monteil, "Karla Sofía Gascón Becomes the First Trans Performer to Win Best Actress at Cannes," *Them*, May 28, 2024, www.them.us/story/karla-sofia-gascon-first-trans-woman-best-actress-cannes.

Antonia Blyth, "Emilia Pérez's Karla Sofía Gascón Becomes the First Openly Trans Person Ever Nominated for an Acting Oscar," *Deadline*, January 23, 2023, deadline.com/2025/01/karla-sofia-gascon-oscar-nomination-2025-1236263101/.

150   "Review of Documentary: Will & Harper," *The Lies They Tell*, September 28, 2024, the-lies-they-tell.org/2024/09/28/review-of-documentary-will-harper/.

Dr. Joseph Burgo, "Are Trans Rights Activists Victims—Or Bullies?" *Daily Caller*, April 14, 2023, dailycaller.com/2023/04/14/opinion-are-trans-rights-activists-victims-or-bullies-dr-joseph-burgo/.

Sexual component diminishes but desire to be female increases in older AGPs: Ray Blanchard, "Clinical Observations and Systematic Studies of Autogynephilia," *Journal of Sex & Marital Therapy*, 1991, doi.org/10.1080/00926239108404348.

151   Author interview with Dr. Ray Blanchard.

Author interview with Becca.

*Names and other identifying details changed to protect anonymity.

Chapter Eight: Males in Girls' Sports—How Is This Fair?

157   "2018–19 Men's Swimming and Diving: Will Thomas," *University of Pennsylvania Athletics*, pennathletics.com/sports/mens-swimming-and-diving/roster/will-thomas/14590.

Thomas 2018–2019 rankings: John Lohn, "A Look at the Numbers and Times: No Denying the Advantages of Lia Thomas," *Swimming World*, April 5, 2022, www.swimmingworldmagazine.com/news/a-look-at-the-numbers-and-times-no-denying-the-advantages-of-lia-thomas/.

158   Katie Barnes, "Amid Protests, Penn Swimmer Lia Thomas Becomes First Known Transgender Athlete to Win Division I National Championship," *ESPN*, March 17, 2022, www.espn.com/college-sports/story/_/id/33529775/amid-protests-pennsylvania-swimmer-lia-thomas-becomes-first-known-transgender-athlete-win-division-national-championship.

158–168   Author interview with Kim Jones.

159   Kelsey J. Santisteban et al., "Sex Differences in VO2max and the Impact on Endurance-Exercise Performance," *International Journal of Environmental Research and Public Health*, April 2022, doi.org/10.3390/ijerph19094946.

Sandro Bartolomei et al., "A Comparison between Male and Female Athletes in Relative Strength and Power Performances," *Journal of Functional Morphology and Kinesiology*, 2021, doi.org/10.3390/jfmk6010017.

"See the Skeletal Differences Between Women and Men," *Human Kinetics*, us.humankinetics.com/blogs/excerpt/see-the-skeletal-differences-between-women-and-men.

160   Lohn, "A Look at the Numbers and Times."

161   *Name changed to protect privacy.

162   Sarah Pruitt, "How Title IX Transformed Women's Sports," *History.com*, June 11, 2021, www.history.com/news/title-nine-womens-sports.

164–168 Author interview with Marshi Smith.

165 *Trophy for tied race given to Lia Thomas:* Ryan Glasspiegal, "Riley Gaines Slams NCAA for 'Trying to Save Face' in Lia ThomasTtie," *NY Post*, April 4, 2022, nypost.com/2022/04/04/swimmer-who-tied-lia-thomas-taken-aback-in-trophy-handling/.

167 Tinbete Ermyas and Kira Wakeam, "Wave of Bills to Block Trans Athletes Has No Basis in Science, Researcher Says," *NPR*, March 18, 2021, www.npr.org/2021/03/18/978716732/wave-of-new-bills-say-trans-athletes-have-an-unfair-edge-what-does-the-science-s.

The male performance advantage: Emma N. Hilton & Tommy R. Lundberg, "Transgender Women in the Female Category of Sport: Perspectives on Testosterone Suppression and Performance Advantage" *Sports Medicine*, 2021, doi.org/10.1007/s40279-020-01389-3.

Doriane Lambelet Coleman and Wickliffe Shreve, "Comparing Athletic Performances the Best Elite WOmen to Boys and Men," *Duke Law*, undated, web.law.duke.edu/sites/default/files/centers/sportslaw/comparingathleticperformances.pdf.

168 Diamy Wang, "Penn Nominates Transgender Swimmer Lia Thomas for NCAA Woman of the Year," *Daily Pennsylvanian*, July 20, 2022, www.thedp.com/article/2022/07/lia-thomas-ncaa-swimming-award-nominated-penn-graduated-transgender.

Author interview with Grace Ellison (pseudonym).

Evan Lips, "Bearded MA 'Trans' HS Athlete Injures Multiple Girls; Now Story Part of NH Debate," *NH Journal*, April 4, 2024, nhjournal.com/bearded-ma-trans-hs-athlete-injures-multiple-girls-now-story-part-of-nh-debate/.

Luke Gentile, "Watch: Transgender Rugby Player Slams Female Athletes, Coach Says Three Injured," *Washington Examiner*, April 14, 2022, www.washingtonexaminer.com/news/1065633/watch-transgender-rugby-player-slams-female-athletes-coach-says-three-injured/.

169 Chelsea Mitchell, "I Was the Fastest Girl in Connecticut. But Transgender Athletes Made It an Unfair Fight, *USA Today*, May 22, 2021, www.usatoday.com/story/opinion/2021/05/22/transgender-athletes-girls-women-sports-track-connecticut-column/5149532001/?gnt-cfr=1&gca-cat=p.

Matt Lavietes, "Transgender Teen Booed after Winning Girls' Track Race at State Championship," *NBC News*, May 21, 2024, www.nbc-news.com/nbc-out/out-news/transgender-teen-booed-winning-girls-track-race-state-championship-rcna153383.

Amanda Roley, "Controversy Arises after Transgender East Valley Student Wins State Track Championship," *KREM2 News*, May 29, 2024, www.krem.com/article/news/local/east-valley-transgender-teen-wins-state-track-controversey/293-2120ce14-825c-46a6-b52e-2f57dedbac55.

Blake and Travis Allen's suspensions and settlement: Mary Margaret Olohan, "Vermont School District Suspends Father of Girl Who Pushed Back Against Biological Male in Her Locker Room, *Daily Signal,* October 18, 2022, www.dailysignal.com/2022/10/18/vermont-school-district-suspends-father-of-girl-who-pushed-back-against-biological-male-in-her-locker-room/.

170   Ray Blanchard, PhD, "Early History of the Concept of Autogynephilia," *Archives of Sexual Behavior,"* August 2005, doi:10.1007/s10508-005-4343-8.

171   Bailey and Blanchard, "Gender Dysphoria Is Not One Thing."

Melissa Koenig, "50-Year-Old Trans Swimmer Shared Locker Room While Competing Against Teens: 'The Girls Were Terrified,'" *New York Post*, December 15, 2023, nypost.com/2023/12/15/news/50-year-old-transgender-woman-shared-pool-locker-room-with-young-girls-at-race/.

172   Author interview with Grace Ellison (pseudonym).

172–175   Author interview with Bridget.

*Names and other identifying details changed.

Chapter Nine: Why Are We Letting Males Invade Female-Only Spaces?

176–184   "Report of the Special Grand Jury on the Investigation of Loudoun Public Schools," including attachments and exhibits, Circuit Court of Loudoun County, Case No. CL-22-3129, December 2022.

179   *Rape not taken seriously generally and rape kits pile up:* Erin Gordon, "Untested Rape Kits: Delays, Destruction, and Disregarded Victims," *American Bar Association,* May 17, 2019, www.americanbar.org/groups/diversity/women/publications/perspectives/2018/may/untested-rape-kits-delays-destruction-and-disregarded-victims/.

Ziegler says no assaults have occurred in school bathrooms: "LCPS School Board and Superintendent Lie to the Citizens of Loudoun," video uploaded by Fight For Schools, October 12, 2021, www.youtube.com/watch?v=Qzk20JwQk2I.

179–182   *Full video, June 22, 2021 Loudoun County School Board meeting:* "Live Re-Feed, Chaotic Loudoun County School Board Meeting, June 22,

2021," video uploaded by The KineticTV, June 22, 2021, www.youtube. com/watch?v=SnU1xzqjZPw.

183   "Loudoun County Teenager Sentenced for 2 Sex Assaults, Must Register as Sex Offender," *FOX 5 DC*, January 12, 2022, www.youtube. com/watch?v=C8cKCxxM5ww.

DA continued to prosecute father of first raped teen: Alex Hammer, "Judge Removes DA from Case of Dad Whose Daughter Was Raped by Trans Boy at School," *Daily Mail*, September 13, 2022, www.dailymail. co.uk/news/article-11208597/Judge-removes-DA-case-dad-daughter-raped-trans-boy-school.html.

NSBA asks White House to investigate parents at school meetings: Carolyn Thompson, "School Board Group Asks US for Help Policing Threats," *Associated Press*, October 1, 2021, smdp.com/news/school-board-group-asks-us-for-help-policing-threats.

"Governor Glenn Youngkin Grants Pardon to Loudoun County Dad Whose Daughter was Sexually Assaulted in Public School," press release, *Office of the Governor Glenn Youngkin of Virginia*, September 10, 2023, www.governor.virginia.gov/newsroom/news-releases/2023/september/name-1013859-en.html.

184   Shawn Cohen, "Exclusive: It Was the Woke Cover-up That Electrified the Virginia Governor's Race, Now on Election Day the Mother of Skirt-Wearing Teen Who Raped a Female Classmate in Girls' Bathroom Says He Is a Troubled Boy Who Identifies as Male and Just Wanted Sex," *Daily Mail*, updated December 7, 2022, www.dailymail. co.uk/news/article-10156749/Mother-skirt-wearing-teen-raped-female-classmate-says-identifies-male.html.

185   Michael Ruiz, "California Trans Child Molester Hannah Tubbs Was Accused of Attacking 4-Year-Old Girl in 2013: Documents," *Fox News*, April 26, 2022, www.foxnews.com/us/california-trans-child-molester-hannah-tubbs-4-year-old-girl-library.

186   "Convicted LA Sex Offender Pleads No Contest to Manslaughter, Father Convicted as Accessory," *BakersfieldNow*, November 8, 2023, bakersfieldnow.com/news/local/convicted-la-sex-offender-pleads-no-contest-to-manslaughter-father-convicted-as-accessory-kern-county-district-attorneys-office-lake-isabella-kern-county-los-angeles-county.

Michael Ruiz, "Trans Child Molester Hannah Tubbs Crafted New Female Identity in Jailhouse Call with Dad, Sources Say," *Fox News*, February 27, 2023, www.foxnews.com/us/trans-child-molester-hannah-tubbs-crafted-new-female-identity-jailhouse-call-dad-sources-say.

Matthew Ormseth, "Adult Who, at 17, Sexually Assaulted Child Is Sentenced to Juvenile Facility," January 27, 2022, www.latimes.com/california/story/2022-01-27/26-year-old-who-sexually-assaulted-girl-while-underage-will-serve-two-year-term-in-juvenile-facility-judge-rules.

187   Michael Ruiz and Bill Melugin, "LA DA Gascón Suspends Prosecutor or Misgendering and 'Deadnaming' Trans Child Molester Accused of Murder," *Fox News*, February 24, 2023, www.foxnews.com/us/la-da-gascon-suspends-prosecutor-misgendering-deadnaming-trans-child-molester-accused-murder.

Michael Ruiz, "Trans Child Molester Sentenced for Killing Friend with a Rock in Fight over $100, *Fox News*, December 8, 2023, www.foxnews.com/us/trans-child-molester-sentenced-killing-friend-rock-fight-over-100.

187–188 Dr. Ian J. Gargan, CPsychol, AFBPsS, "Written Evidence Submitted by British Psychological Society to the Transgender Equality Inquiry," August 20, 2015, data.parliament.uk/WrittenEvidence/CommitteeEvidence.svc/EvidenceDocument/Women%20and%20Equalities/Transgender%20Equality/written/19471.html.

189   "United Kingdom: Scotland," World Prison Brief, www.prisonstudies.org/country/united-kingdom-scotland.

189   *Most males in Scotland's prisons who claimed to be trans only did so after conviction:* Georgina Cutler, "Scotland's Trans Prisoner Shame: More Than 60 Per cent Began Transitioning after Being Convicted," *GB News,* March 28, 2023, www.gbnews.com/news/scotland-trans-prisoners-transition-after-conviction-snp-gender-reforms.

"Isla Bryson: Transgender Rapist Jailed for Eight Years," *BBC*, February 28, 2023, www.bbc.com/news/uk-scotland-64796926.

Brad Hunter, "Study Finds Nearly 45% of Trans-Women Inmates Convicted of Sex Crimes," *Toronto Sun*, February 1, 2023, torontosun.com/news/national/study-finds-nearly-45-of-trans-women-inmates-convicted-of-sex-crimes.

190   President Donald Trump, "Defending Women from Gender Ideology Extremism and Restoring Biological Truth to the Federal Government," Executive Order, January 20, 2025, www.whitehouse.gov/presidential-actions/2025/01/defending-women-from-gender-ideology-extremism-and-restoring-biological-truth-to-the-federal-government/.

Statistics on US prisoners incarcerated for sex crimes: "Offenses," *Federal Bureau of Prisons*, www.bop.gov/about/statistics/statistics_inmate_offenses.jsp (last updated July 2025).

Anna Slatz, "USA: Almost 50% of Trans Inmates in Federal Custody for Sex Offences," *4th Wave*, January 3, 2022, 4w.pub/50-of-trans-inmates-in-federal-custody-for-sex-offences/.

Anna Slatz, "Trans-Identified Male Who Murdered His Girlfriend Deemed 'Vulnerable' by Oregon Court, Seeking Transfer to Women's Prison," *Reduxx*, September 11, 2023, reduxx.info/trans-male-who-murdered-his-girlfriend-deemed-vulnerable-by-oregon-court-seeking-transfer-to-womens-prison/.

191   Genevieve Gluck, "Sadistic Killer with a 'Blood Fetish' Transferred to NJ Women's Prison," *Reduxx*, April 14, 2022, reduxx.info/sadistic-killer-with-a-blood-fetish-transferred-to-nj-womens-prison/.

Joe Atmonavage, "Two Women at N.J. Prison Are Pregnant after Consensual Sex Between Inmates, DOC Says," *NJ.com*, April 13, 2022, www.nj.com/news/2022/04/two-women-at-nj-prison-are-pregnant-after-consensual-sex-between-inmates-doc-says.html.

Matt Masterson, "Lawsuit: Female Prisoner Says She Was Raped by Transgender Inmate," *WTTW*, February 19, 2020, news.wttw.com/2020/02/19/lawsuit-female-prisoner-says-she-was-raped-transgender-inmate.

@ACLU post on Owen execution, June 16, 2023, https://x.com/ACLU/status/1669705153316880385.

Psychiatrists said Owens faked gender ID, schizophrenia, and dementia: "Florida Executes Duane Owen for 1984 Killings of Teenage Babysitter and Mother of 2," *CBS News*, June 16, 2023, www.cbsnews.com/news/florida-executes-duane-owen-1984-killings-karen-slattery-georgianna-worden/.

192   Mary Kate Leming, "Should 'Mental Illness' Spare Owen from Execution?" *Coastal Star*, March 5, 2015, thecoastalstar.com/profiles/blogs/should-mental-illness-spare-owen-from-execution.

"Incels (Involuntary Celibates)," *Anti-Defamation League*, July 11, 2025, www.adl.org/resources/backgrounder/incels-involuntary-celibates (last updated).

193   Jennifer Gingrich, "Georgia Man Arrested after Exposing Himself to 15-Year-Old Girl in Planet Fitness Locker Room," *Reduxx*, September 21, 2023, reduxx.info/georgia-man-arrested-after-exposing-himself-to-15-year-old-girl-in-planet-fitness-locker-room/.

Chapter Ten: Why Have We All Gone Mad?

195   *Leslie Elliot's grad school enforces social justice ideas:* Ethan Blevins, "Must an Antioch Student Bow Down to 'Social Justice' Dogma to Graduate?" *Hill,* February 6, 2023, thehill.com/opinion/education/3844048-must-an-antioch-student-bow-down-to-social-justice-dogma-to-graduate/.

196   *Training for social workers expects critical social justice ideology mindset:* "2024 Standards Glossary," CACREP, www.cacrep.org/2024-standards-glossary-2/.
       Author interview with David Habib Martin.

197   *English curriculum:* "Literature & Social Justice Mission Statement," LeHigh University Department of English, undated, english.cas.lehigh.edu/literature-social-justice/mission-statement.
       Philosophy curriculum and social justice: "Philosophy . . . Social Justice Track," Wesleyan University, www.wesleyan.edu/philosophy/about_major.html.
       Medical school social justice warriors: Travis J. Morrell, "Ideology in Medical Schools Threatens Everyone's Health," *Wall Street Journal,* July 26, 2024, www.wsj.com/articles/ideology-in-medical-schools-threatens-everyones-health-f6887ae3.
       Ryan General, "Vanderbilt Professor Says Math Education Is Too 'White, Cisheteropatriarchal,'" *Yahoo News,* January 27, 2023, www.yahoo.com/news/vanderbilt-professor-says-math-education-200027972.html.

198   Amanda MacGregor, "To Teach or Not to Teach: Is Shakespeare Still Relevant to Today's Students?" *School Library Journal,* January 4, 2021, www.slj.com/story/to-teach-or-not-to-teach-is-shakespeare-still-relevant-to-todays-students-libraries-classic-literature-canon.
       Claims that historical queens and Joan of Arc were trans/non-binary: Dr. Kit Heyam, "'It Was Necessary': Taking Joan of Arc on Their Own Terms," *Shakespeare's Globe,* August 2022, www.shakespearesglobe.com/discover/blogs-and-features/2022/08/08/it-was-necessary-taking-joan-of-arc-on-their-own-terms/.
       Experience Biology (Savvas Learning Company 2020).
       Lisa A. Urry et al., *AP Campbell Biology in Focus,* 3rd edition (Pearson March 2019).
       Letter to "Let's Talk About Sex, Baby," anthropology conference panel: Ramona Perez, president, AAA, and Monica Heller, president, CASCA, American Anthropological Association, September 25, 2023.

199   Emily Drabinski, "Queering the Catalog: Queer Theory and the Politics of Correction," *Library Quarterly*, April 2013, doi.org/10.1086/669547.

Daniel Payne, "Mexican High Court Finds Ex-Congressman Guilty of 'Gender-Based Political Violence' Over Tweet," *National Catholic Register*, August 10, 2023, www.ncregister.com/cna/mexican-high-court-finds-ex-congressman-guilty-of-gender-based-political-vio-lence-over-tweet.

Nuria Muíña García, "Spain: Trans-Identified Male Sentenced to Six Months in Prison after Making 'Transphobic' Comments Towards Another Trans-Identified Male for Not Having Genital Surgery," *Reduxx*, February 21, 2024, reduxx.info/spain-man-sentenced-to-six-months-in-prison-after-making-transphobic-comments-towards-male-ex-prostitute/.

"Surrey Police Investigation over 'Misgendering' Tweets," *BBC*, March 20, 2019, www.bbc.com/news/uk-england-surrey-47638527.

NYC law against misgendering: NYC Human Rights Law, Title 8 of the Administrative Code of the City of New York, www.nyc.gov/site/cchr/law/text-of-the-law.page.

Naaman Zhou, "'We Deserve the Dignity of Being Known': Teddy Cook's Transgender Speech to NSW Parliament Praised," *Guardian*, April 23, 2021, www.theguardian.com/society/2021/apr/23/we-de-serve-the-dignity-of-being-known-teddy-cooks-transgender-speech-to-nsw-parliament-praised.

Max Aitchison, "Why This 'Disparaging' Post about an Aussie UN Trans Expert Who Plugs Bondage, Bestiality, Drugs, and Taxpay-er-Funded Sex-Change Ops MUST Be Taken Down—or Billion-aire Elon Musk Will Cop an $800,000 Fine," *Daily Mail Australia*, March 26, 2024, www.dailymail.co.uk/news/article-13239427/X-eS-afety-Commissioner-trans-Teddy-Cook.html.

200   *Portland Public Schools sex ed:* @realchrisrufo, post on X, July 27, 2022, x.com/realchrisrufo/status/1552397094593277953.

201   Author correspondence with representatives of Portland Public Schools.

202   George M. Johnson, *All Boys Aren't Blue* (Farrar, Strauss & Giroux 2020).

Susan Kuklin, *Beyond Magenta* (Candlewick 2014).

Maia Kobabe, *Gender Queer* (Oni Press 2019).

Juno Dawson, *This Book Is Gay* (Sourcebooks Fire 2021).

Erika Moen and Matthew Nolan, *Let's Talk About It* (Random House Graphic 2021).

203–204 *Be Ready, Be Real* (San Francisco Unified School District 2017).

204 Author interview with Lisa Mullins.

205 Author interview with Alesha Perkins.

Author correspondence with Portland Public Schools representative.

205–208 "District-wide K–12 Health Curriculum," Portland Public Schools, www.pps.net/Page/16164 (last accessed July 15, 2025).

208 Marielena Meder, "AUSTRIA: Children Expelled from Kindergarten after Their Parents Objected to Poster Depicting Naked Trans-Identified Male Displaying His Penis," *Reduxx*, January 9, 2025, reduxx. info/austria-children-expelled-from-kindergarten-after-their-parents-objected-to-poster-depicting-naked-trans-identified-male-displaying-his-penis/.

Planned Parenthood's Teen Council (Washington state), "Puberty."

"Taiwanese Parents Outraged after Gender Identity Survey Given to Schoolchildren Asks Whether They've Taken Lewd Photos of Themselves, *Reduxx*, January 6, 2025, reduxx.info/taiwanese-parents-outraged-after-gender-identity-survey-given-to-schoolchildren-asks-whether-theyve-taken-photos-of-their-genitalia/.

208–212 Author interview with Derrick Jensen.

209 "Queer Theory Jeopardy!!! with Professor Derrick Jensen," video uploaded by Port Film Co-op, September 17, 2020, www.youtube.com/watch?v=n-NseFg2kno.

210 Meredith Evans, "Who Is Alok Vaid-Menon, Sam Smith's and Demi Lovato's Alleged 'Handler' Who May Have Influenced Them to Be Non-Binary and Called Little Girls 'Kinky'?" *Evie*, March 21, 2023, www.eviemagazine.com/post/who-is-alok-vaid-menon-sam-smith-demi-lovatos-handler-nonbinary.

See the Amazon listing for Derrick Jensen, *Anarchism and the Politics of Violation* (Seven Stories Press, January 2, 2079), www.amazon.com/gp/product/1609808770/.

212 Jennifer Bilek, "The Billionaire Family Pushing Synthetic Sex Identities (SSI)," *Tablet Magazine*, June 14, 2022, www.tabletmag.com/sections/news/articles/billionaire-family-pushing-synthetic-sex-identities-ssi-pritzkers.

213 *Pritzker family fortune:* "Pritzker Family," *Wikipedia*, en.wikipedia.org/wiki/Pritzker_family (last accessed September 2023).

214 *Average costs of vaginoplasty and phalloplasty:* Baker K, Restar A., "Utilization and Costs of Gender-Affirming Care in a Commercially Insured Transgender Population," *Journal of Law and Medical Ethics*, 2022, doi: 10.1017/jme.2022.87; "How Much Does Testosterone HRT Cost at

Folx?" *Folx*, August 1, 2023, www.folxhealth.com/library/how-much-does-testosterone-hrt-cost-at-folx.

Chapter Eleven: It's Time to Reclaim Reality and Sanity

216   Gayle S. Rubin, "Thinking Sex: Notes for a Radical Theory of the Politics of Sexuality," in *Pleasure and Danger: Exploring Female Sexuality*, ed. Carol S. Vance (Routledge & Kegan Paul 1984), 143–179.
       G.K. Chesterton, *The Thing* (S&W January 1929).

217   *Seattle naked guy in rainbow legwarmers:* @MACdivasenoRITA, post on X, x.com/MACdivasenoRITA/status/1834384696618483747 (last accessed September 13, 2024). See also: "Nudist," Reddit r/Seattle, www.reddit.com/r/Seattle/comments/1fc9e82/nudist/ (last accessed September 13, 2024).

217–218 *Middle-Schoolers Told to Google "Penises and Vaginas":* Author interviews with students and parents who requested anonymity.

218   *Indiana male murderer IDs as Muslim, Wiccan woman:* Sarah Loesch Jon Webb, "Judge Sides with Evansville Transgender Woman Seeking Gender-Affirming Surgery in Prison," *Evansville Courier & Press*, September 20, 2024, www.courierpress.com/story/news/local/2024/09/20/judge-sides-with-transgender-inmate-seeking-gender-affirming-surgery/75305308007/.
       Victoria, Australia prison for non-affirming parents: "About the Act," Victoria Equal Opportunity & Human Rights Commission, www.humanrights.vic.gov.au/change-or-suppression-practices/about-the-csp-act/.
       Adult nursery in Blaydon, England: @TullipR, post on X, x.com/TullipR/status/1836144174581641217 (last accessed 2024).
       David Cazan, "French Gynaecologist Suspended for Refusing to Treat Trans Woman," *Times*, January 31, 2025, www.thetimes.com/world/europe/article/french-gynaecologist-suspended-for-refusing-to-treat-trans-woman-ldtcjtsbz#Echobox=1738342620.
       Balenciaga's fetish teddy bears: "Balenciaga Campaign: Kim Kardashian 'Shaken' by Fashion House Shoot," *BBC*, www.bbc.com/news/newsbeat-63779620.
       Bryndís Blackadder, "Exclusive: Midwifery Students Taught How to Care for Males Giving Birth," *Reduxx*, April 27, 2022, reduxx.info/exclusive-midwifery-students-taught-how-to-care-for-males-giving-birth/.

219   Nuria Muíña García, "Spain: Trans-Identified Male Sentenced to Six
            Months in Prison after Making 'Transphobic' Comments Towards
            Another Trans-Identified Male for Not Having Genital Surgery,"
            Reduxx, February 21, 2024, eduxx.info/spain-man-sentenced-to-six-
            months-in-prison-after-making-transphobic-comments-towards-
            male-ex-prostitute/.
            Canada's Online Harms Act: "Bill C-63: An Act to Enact the Online
            Harms Act, to Amend the Criminal Code, the Canadian Human
            Rights Act and an Act Respecting the Mandatory Reporting of Inter-
            net Child Pornography by Persons Who Provide an Internet Service
            and to Make Consequential and Related Amendments to Other Acts,"
            Department of Justice, Canada, date modified June 4, 2024, www.jus-
            tice.gc.ca/eng/csj-sjc/pl/charter-charte/c63.html.

219–220   *Hannah Ulrey: Ulery v. Rafferty, MD et al.*, Case Number: PC-2023-
            05366, Providence/Bristol County Superior Court, amended com-
            plaint, October 23, 2023.

220   *Expanded statute of limitations for disability, including mental incompe-
            tence:* Christie Nicholson, JD, "Rhode Island Civil Statute of Limita-
            tions Law," *Findlaw*, April 4, 2025, www.findlaw.com/state/rhode-is-
            land-law/rhode-island-civil-statute-of-limitations-laws.html. See also
            webserver.rilin.state.ri.us/Statutes/title9/9-1/9-1-14.3.HTM.
            "State Medical Malpractice Laws, Lawsuit-Filing Deadlines,
            and Damages Caps," *Nolo*, www.nolo.com/legal-encyclopedia/
            state-state-medical-malpractice-statute-limitations (last accessed July
            2025).

221   Author interview with Robert Weisenburger.

222   "Rising Malpractice Premiums Push Small Clinics Away from Gen-
            der-Affirming Care for Minors," *PBS News Hour*, January 20, 2024,
            www.pbs.org/newshour/health/rising-malpractice-premiums-push-
            small-clinics-away-from-gender-affirming-care-for-minors.
            President Donald Trump, "Protecting Children from Chemical
            and Surgical Mutilation," Executive Order, January 28, 2025, www.
            whitehouse.gov/presidential-actions/2025/01/protecting-chil-
            dren-from-chemical-and-surgical-mutilation/.
            Montana statute of limitations law update: "MT HB 682," *Bill Track
            50*, signed into law May 13, 2025, www.billtrack50.com/billde-
            tail/1750076/multi-collapse.

224–225   *Judge calls teaching gender ideology "religious views": Mirabelli v. Olson*,
            "Order Denying Defendants' Motions to Dismiss," Case 3:23-cv-
            00768-BEN-VET, Document 194, January 7, 2025, 21–22.

225   *PFLAG sues on First Amendment grounds: PFLAG et al. v. Donald J. Trump et al.*, Case 1:25-cv-00337-BAH, Document 1, filed February 2, 2025.
Kara Dansky, "These Lawsuits!" *Terf Report*, February 14, 2025, kara-dansky.substack.com/p/these-lawsuits.

226   Jillian Smith, "Poll: Majority of Americans Oppose Instruction on Gender Identity for Young Students," *CBS News Austin,* September 20, 2022, cbsaustin.com/news/nation-world/poll-majority-of-amer-icans-oppose-instruction-on-sex-gender-identity-for-young-stu-dents-gov-glenn-youngkin-ron-desantis-parents-defending-educa-tion-new-york-times-poll-70-of-americans-opposed-to-teaching-about-sexual-orientation-gender-identity-lgbtq.
Moms For Liberty, www.momsforliberty.org/.

227   *Journalists who question child gender "transitions" but refer to adults by the wrong pronouns:* Ben Ryan, "Why I Use Trans People's Preferred Pro-nouns," *Hazard Ratio: Benjamin Ryan,* February 25, 2025, benryan.sub-stack.com/p/why-i-use-trans-peoples-preferred. See also: *Helen Lewis calls Chase Strangio, "he":* Helen Lewis, "The Liberal Misinformation Bubble about Youth Gender Medicine," *Atlantic,* June 29, 2025, www.theatlantic.com/ideas/archive/2025/06/transgender-youth-skrmet-ti/683350/?gift=KkbsgAqgmImeUM71Y0bfDPq00DkEVN3jlt2g-pN_8uhc. See also: *Andrew Sullivan calls males "she":* Andrew Sullivan, "Rachel Levine Must Resign," *The Weekly Dish,* October 18, 2024, sub-stack.com/home/post/p-150390017.

228   Anita Bartholomew, "To My Dear Friends: No, I Don't Believe Your Son Is Now Your Daughter," *Good Question,* December 2, 2024, anit-abartholomew.substack.com/p/to-my-dear-friends-no-i-dont-believe.
Christina Farmer et al., "A Review of Academic Use of the Term 'Mi-nor Attracted Persons,'" *Trauma, Violence, Abuse,* September 15, 2024, doi:10.1177/15248380241270028.
Michael Bailey, PhD, on "virtuous pedophiles": Screenshot posted by @DuncanHenry78, September 19, 2024, of a deleted post on X by @profjmb dated February 27, 2024, x.com/DuncanHenry78/sta-tus/1836828694075298088.

Appendix I: The Effects and Limits of Trump's Executive Orders

232–234   Author interview with Kara Danksy.
232   President Donald Trump, "Defending Women from Gender Ideology

Extremism and Restoring Biological Truth to the Federal Government," Executive Order, January 20, 2025.

"Biden Administration's Final Title IX Rule Goes Into Effect Aug. 1," American Council on Education, April 22, 2024, www.acenet.edu/News-Room/Pages/Biden-Admin-Final-Title-IX-Rule-Effective-Aug-1.aspx.

About the Author

Anita Bartholomew is a former longtime contributing editor and contributor to both the US and international editions of *Reader's Digest*, where she covered topics spanning health, science, social issues, and politics. She is the author of *Siege: An American Tragedy*, a detailed account of the storming of the US Capitol on January 6, 2021, and the co-author of the critically acclaimed award-winning medical memoir: *Something to Prove: A Daughter's Journey to Fulfill a Father's Legacy*. In connection with her reporting, she's appeared as a guest on TV news, true crime, and talk shows. Two of her long-form narratives have been adapted for TV films. She lives in Oregon.